Healthy Teas

green • black • herbal • fruit

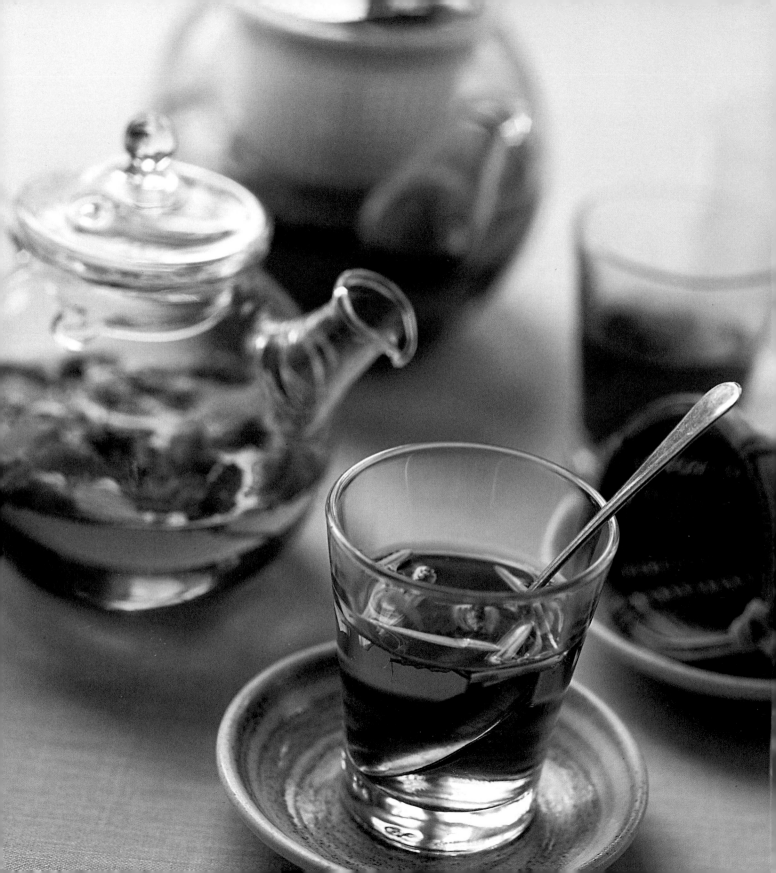

Healthy Teas

green • black • herbal • fruit

Tammy Safi

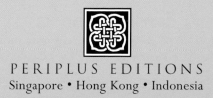

PERIPLUS EDITIONS

Singapore • Hong Kong • Indonesia

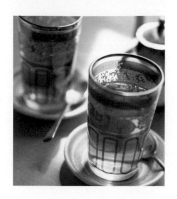

Contents

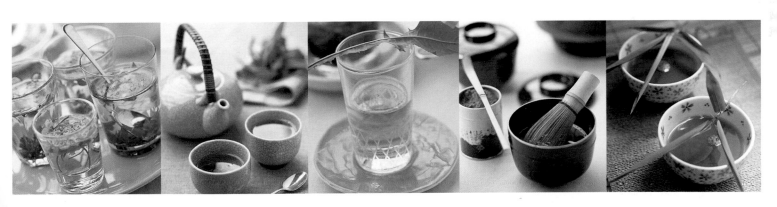

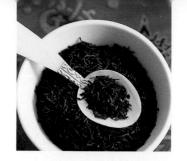

Recipes

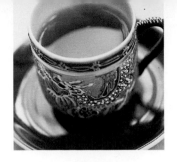

INTRODUCTION

My love for tea started years ago. When I was a child, my father would brew a strong, milky, sweet tea for both of us. As he was pouring it, he would ask, "One or two teaspoons, Tammy?" My answer was always two, but he asked, nevertheless. The time we spent sipping a cup of tea was our time. We still sit and drink tea together, but today the tea is more likely to be lemon grass or cinnamon. My father continues to ask, "Any sugar, Tammy?" Even though I always reply, "No thanks, Dad. No sugar," he asks every time.

Now a qualified herbalist and nutritionist, my interest in the therapeutic properties of plants and herbs also started many years ago, when I lived in Lebanon. My newborn baby suffered from colic, and one morning my nosy neighbor heard him screaming. She barged her way into my kitchen—as she always did—with a handful of sweet-smelling seeds. I watched her infuse the seeds and witnessed my first cup of herb tea: aniseed. The tea worked like magic. My son was soon out of his misery and fast asleep.

In this book I explore tea as we know it today: its origins, where it is grown and cultivated, and how it has been used for thousands of years for both pleasure and medicinal purposes, particularly green tea. The recipes that follow include those that can be used for health and wellbeing, and those that are commonly drunk in Asia, along with some interesting floral and fruit blends.

Tea was my constant companion during the writing of this book, and nothing gives me more pleasure than passing on my knowledge of this delectable brew. Most of the ingredients in this book are readily available at supermarkets, natural foods stores, or Asian, Indian, and Lebanese grocery stores, or Chinese herb stores. However, it is well worth growing your own herbs. There is nothing like the fragrance of freshly cut lavender or yarrow. If you plant just a few different herbs each month, you will have a herb garden with the most tantalizing aromas before you know it.

ASIAN TEAS:
A WAY OF LIFE

Asians have a great deal of respect for tea. They serve it with every meal to help facilitate digestion. It is also served to guests as a warm welcoming beverage. The tea plant, *Camellia sinensis*, is a beautiful evergreen native to Southeast Asia. It is grown mostly in China, India, Indonesia, Sri Lanka and Japan. It grows best in the mountains, far above sea level, where the days are sunny, the nights rainy and the air clean and fresh. The best green teas are grown at 5000 feet (1525 meters) above sea level.

It's All in the Process

Plantation pickers rise before sunrise and spend the day expertly picking the precious leaves with just a swift flick of their fingers. When a basket is full, it is returned to the factory; the leaves then undergo a number of delicate and important stages before the tea is ready to brew. These processes include:

Fermentation: The leaves are kept in a moist 72°–82°F (30°C) atmosphere so that they warm up and then begin to cool. If the temperature is any higher, the tea will be tainted with a burnt taste. Any lower, and the fermentation process will stop. Fermentation ends just before the leaves begin to cool. This can take one to three hours. The leaves are then dried in machines at 175°F (80°C) for twenty minutes. If the tea is fired for too long, the leaves will lose their flavor. On the other hand, if they are not fired long enough, mold will form.

Withering: Tea leaves are spread over screens or woven straw mats, which are then stacked on top of each other so that warm air can circulate around the leaves, ensuring that mold doesn't form. They are left to dry for 24 hours, after which the leaves are crisp and completely dry.

Pan-firing: This method is usually reserved for the production of green tea. The leaves are constantly stirred in woks over a consistent heat until they are dry.

Steaming: This method is usually used in Japan for green-tea production. The tea leaves are steamed in trays over boiling water to soften them and prevent oxidation.

Rolling: This can be done by hand or machine, and it is a method usually reserved for green tea. The tea leaves are rolled into curls, twists, and other shapes, which affect the flavor during infusion.

Naming Teas

Teas of the world are classified in a number of ways. One is by the size and shape of the processed leaf. Another is by the way it is processed. Tea leaves are grouped by hand. Traditional manufacturing yields a large leaf with smaller broken pieces, or grades. The leaves are spread over mats according to whether they are whole or broken, as well as according to their size. The leaves are named according to their length: "dust" is less than 0.04 inch (1 mm) in length, and "fanning" is less than 0.06 inch (1.5 mm).

Another way of classifying a tea is by the country or district where it is grown, such as China, India, Ceylon, or Japan.

Different teas work best at different times, depending on what you are doing and your state of health. In Asia, each tea is drunk for its own specific effect and taste. Black tea has a significant amount of caffeine, is warming, and acts as a digestive, while green tea is cooling and cleansing, with low amounts of caffeine. Black tea is often drunk in the morning or when you need a boost, but because green tea helps to reduce cholesterol by lowering blood lipids, it is best drunk with meals or with a sweet between meals.

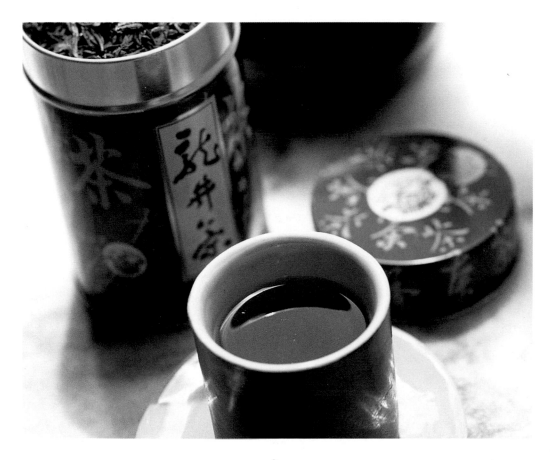

THE HISTORY OF ASIAN TEAS

Tea is made by steeping or boiling chopped plant material—roots, leaves, and flowers—for a specified amount of time. It is a warm, soothing drink that brings to mind good company, good times and happy days. The art of making the humble cup of tea has been lovingly passed down through the generations for thousands of centuries.

Chinese Origins

Tea is believed to have originated in China in 2737BC. Legend has it that Emperor Sh'eng Nung was spending a day in the countryside. He was sipping a cup of hot water, as was his custom, when a few leaves from a tree blew into the cup. The aroma from the mix was so enticing that he sipped the brew and a new beverage was born. Since then, there has been a lot of experimenting with boiling water and the leaf of that evergreen, *Camellia sinensis*.

During the Sung Dynasty, 960–1279AD, tea making was considered an art form. As tea was rare and costly, affordable only by the elite, competitions would take place among royal families to determine who could perfect the most skillful techniques for making tea. These competitions made tea a highly desired beverage. Before long, its use spread and green tea became the most popular of all.

Many provinces created distinctive methods of brewing. The Fujian province, for example, rolled tea leaves into a ball. Pieces were scraped off these balls and then placed in a glazed bowl. Hot water was added and the mixture was stirred until a white froth formed. The longer the froth lasted, the better. The liquid tea, however, had to be clear.

Picked in India

Tea is believed to have been introduced into India around 500AD by Siddhartha, the prince who became the Buddha. It is said that Siddhartha left India, pledging to remain awake for nine years in order to meditate and travel for enlightenment. After five years, he was overcome by sleep. While resting beside a green bush, he picked some of its leaves and chewed them. They revived him, giving him alertness and energy. Siddhartha continued his journey with this newfound tea. When he returned to India he brought tea seeds to be planted.

India became the largest tea-growing country when Robert Fortune, a botanist and spy for the East India Company, transported 23,000 young plants and 17,000 seedlings from China to India between 1848 and 1851. Fortune wrote many best-selling books, full of adventure and excitement, about his travels from China to India. The Indians adopted the English practice of serving tea with milk and sugar. They also had their own "local" tea, masala chai, which is a fragrant, sweet, warming tea, made with milk and spices.

Revered in Japan

Dengyo Daishi, a Buddhist monk, is generally credited with bringing tea to Japan after traveling to China around 803–805AD. He did so after he noticed that tea had the ability to keep the monks in China awake and alert during long hours of meditation and prayer.

The first Japanese book about tea is called *The Book Of Tea Sanitation*, by Eisai, a Buddhist monk, and was published in 1211AD. It is also known as *Maintaining Health By Drinking Tea*. In his book, Eisai describes the benefits of drinking tea and how it could be used to treat some illnesses. After this, Japanese monks took tea drinking to a different level, embracing it within their spiritual ceremonies and beliefs.

Tea is thought to have reached the rest of Asia by the end of the sixth century, thanks to Zen Buddhist monks, who traveled widely.

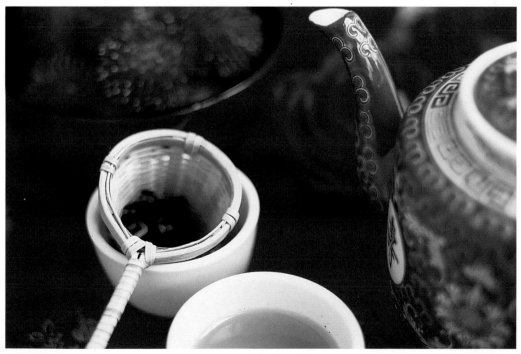

Migrating West

The earliest reference to tea in Europe is in 1559. A Venetian citizen wrote a book called *Voyages and Travels*, which mentions chai catai (tea of China). R.L. Wickham, of the English East India Company, is thought to have been the first to mention tea in England in 1615. Before tea came along, the English drank more coffee than any other nation.

The much-loved Assam tea is believed to have been discovered by Major Robert Bruce, a Scotsman, who found tea bushes growing on both sides of the Brahmaputra River in Assam in 1823. Plantations were soon set up, areas cleared, and the first tea from Assam was auctioned in England in 1839. Assam tea lovers believe that this tea has the strength to cure all weaknesses.

A Coming of Age

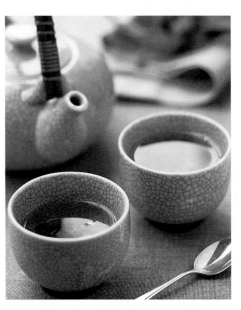

These days, there are hundreds of different grades, qualities, and varieties of tea. Dedicated tea drinkers take tea as seriously as cheese tasters do cheese, or wine connoisseurs wine. And tea has moved beyond the black tea that we first think of to include many other plant ingredients.

Herbs may be more familiar to people as a culinary flavoring. Rosemary, thyme, mint, and sage are common in Western cuisine. But herbs, as well many other plants, including fruits, can be made into teas using either one herb or a mixture of several. You can also add flowers and spices.

Herbal teas are becoming more popular because of their strong medicinal properties. Hippocrates' wise words, "Let your food be your medicine and your medicine be your food," are often quoted for their truth and efficacy, and they are certainly appropriate as far as herbal teas are concerned.

Floral and fruit teas have the added advantage of bringing scent and beauty to a cup of tea. The variety of dried fruits and flowers available, mixed and matched in different combinations, can create a fragrant and attractive beverage to delight family and friends.

If you have a cold, infection, or a feeling of dampness in your body, it is best to drink diaphoretic teas such as ginger and sage. These teas encourage sweating and should be drunk warm or hot until you break out in a sweat. Bitter-tasting teas, such as dandelion, chamomile, and green or jasmine, can enhance digestion and decrease allergic reactions, and they should be drunk before meals. The bitter taste stimulates the flow of digestive juices, preventing bloating and discomfort.

TEA AND YOUR HEALTH

Since ancient times, humans have experimented with nearly every plant and discovered which are safe and which are poisonous. However, it takes a trained herbalist to distinguish between toxic and nontoxic plants.

The Medicinal Use of Plants

Plants are often used to treat a disease or an ailment. For instance, cuts, bruises, and other injuries can be treated with strong anti-inflammatory and quick-healing herbs, such as comfrey (*Symphytum officinale*) or plantain (*Plantago major*) applied as a poultice. Seeds, leaves, stalks, bark, and flowers from a variety of plants and shrubs can be used to treat tummy upsets, fever, dyspepsia, and many other ailments. Plants are also, generally, highly nutritious. They are packed with vitamins, minerals, and other active constituents that can create a positive effect within the body.

The first documentation of the medicinal properties of plants dates back to 1578AD when Shih-Chen Li wrote *An Outline Of Materia Medica*. The Yellow Emperor's *Classics of Internal Medicine*, written over two thousand years ago by herbalists in Nei Ching, is another invaluable source of ancient wisdom. Empirical knowledge—knowledge that is based on experience and observation—has also been handed down from generation to generation within many cultures, and this information is priceless.

The writings of Kuo P'o, a famous Chinese scholar who wrote *Erh Ya* (a dictionary dating from 359AD), includes references to boiling medicinal green leaves, then called k'utu.

The Health Benefits of Tea

It is often said in Chinese literature that foods and medicine share a common source. This is almost certainly the case with tea. It has been proven that the strong antioxidants found in tea are anticancerous. This fact may explain why Asians have the lowest rate of heart disease and cancer in the world, despite a high percentage of heavy smokers among the population.

Tea contains tannins, fluoride, selenium, zinc, flavonols, polyphenols, beta-carotene, and vitamins C and E. It also has an alkaline effect within the body. This alkalinity makes it useful in the treatment of ulcers, or for those who eat too many foods that have an acid-forming reaction in the body, such as meats and dairy products.

The Benefits of Green Tea

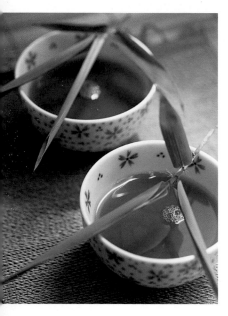

Green tea provides the richest health benefits of all teas. It is the most potent, retaining more vitamins and minerals than other teas. Polyphenols, vitamin E, vitamin C, fluoride, quercetin, tannins, and volatile oils work together as strong antioxidants to help the body ward off carcinogenic mutations. Green tea is cooling and cleansing, with low amounts of caffeine, and is rich in vitamins A, B2, C, D, and E, and flavonoids. Green tea helps to reduce cholesterol by lowering blood lipids.

Scientists have proven over the last fifteen years or so, with experiments on mice, that green tea can both prevent and reduce the incidence of stomach and skin cancers. Green tea is thought to be twenty times stronger than vitamin E in its antiaging properties. It reduces free-radical damage and DNA mutation of cells in the body. Green tea is rich in vitamin C and other antioxidants, such as vitamin E and quercetin. Drinking three to four cups a day of this liquid is worth its weight in gold.

Tannins

Tannins are found in the roots, bark, leaves, and fruit of some plants. They have been used for centuries to tan animal hides in making leather. During the tanning process, tannins and protein come into contact with each other, causing the protein cells to curdle and shrink, tightening the skin.

Tannins are present in black tea and, to a lesser extent, green tea. They are complex polyphenols that have an astringent effect on the body. This astringency causes a tightening and drying of skin and mucous membranes. When you drink a strong cup of black tea, you can gauge the strength of the tannins by the fuzzy feeling on your tongue.

There are good and bad elements to tannins. They can stain the teeth after prolonged tea drinking. They may decrease the absorption of vitamins and minerals, as they can "tan" the stomach lining. They can also aggravate constipation. By adding a squeeze of lemon or a dash of milk to tea, however, you can bind the tannins. Milk and lemon cause the tannins to precipitate, making them less effective. On the positive side, it is the tannins that give tea some of its color and taste. Tannins are also useful to control diarrhea, soothe sore red eyes, and treat infections of the mouth and cervix. To get the maximum amount of tannins from tea, it should be steeped for three to five minutes.

Black tea contains about six to eight percent tannins. Green tea contains negligible amounts. As a result, it can be consumed without milk or lemon and will not cause constipation. Oolong contains about 20 percent tannins. Chinese black tea contains about seven percent, and Indian black tea contains about eight percent. Some herbs also contain tannins, with the highest percentage found in Oak bark, which is prescribed internally to tone and heal mucous membranes for those suffering from diarrhea, and externally for weeping eczema and other skin conditions.

Caffeine

Caffeine is an alkaloid found mainly in tea, coffee, and cola drinks, as well as in chocolate, soft drinks, and "sports" drinks made with guarana, a Brazilian cocoa that contains seven percent caffeine and twelve percent tannins. Caffeine has a bitter taste and acts as a stimulant to the central nervous system.

The stimulating effects of caffeine can be harmful if taken in excess. It can increase blood pressure; urine secretions (by 30 percent); acid secretions, resulting in reflux and inflammation in the stomach; heart rate; and breathing. On the other hand, if used sensibly, caffeine can have positive effects, such as increasing alertness, reducing migraine attacks (due to its ability to constrict dilated blood vessels), and widening bronchial airways in asthmatics if the sufferer is not accustomed to caffeine.

Caffeine can also be addictive. Drinking $1/8$ ounce (350 mg) of caffeine per day, the equivalent of four cups of coffee or eight cups of black tea, is addictive. Drinking the equivalent of a cup of coffee after eating can interfere with the body's absorption of iron and B vitamins. This decrease in the amounts of nutrients absorbed by the body can increase blood cholesterol and cause insomnia. Pregnant woman who drink $1/4$ ounce (650 mg) of caffeine per day can cause serious DNA changes in their unborn child, leading to mutations and defects. The baby may also be born with caffeine dependency.

The caffeine and phosphates in soft drinks flush calcium from bones. Women with menopausal symptoms of bone loss and irritability should totally avoid all products containing caffeine.

Tea contains only half the amount of caffeine that coffee does. The caffeine in tea is known as theophylline and theobromine, which are much milder and gentler stimulants than the caffeine found in coffee and have fewer side effects.

Methods of Brewing

The best tea is made from organically grown plants. The leaves, flowers, roots, or bark should crackle when dry. Tea bags don't usually produce as good a result as loose tea. When buying tea, you can distinguish a good tea leaf from a poor-quality one by smelling it to make sure that there is no mold present and that the tea has a full aroma. Most of the recipes in this book can be made either directly in the cup or in a teapot. Ceramic or glass teapots are preferable, as these materials do not interfere with the flavor of the tea.

The ingredients used to make tea can be bought fresh, dried, or in a powdered form. Some recipes in this book call for the fresh plant to be used. If it is not available, use the dried substitute. **When brewing, bear in mind that, generally, 1 teaspoon of freshly chopped herbs ("herb" refers to the flower, leaf or stem) equals** $1/2$ **teaspoon of the herb dried, or** $1/4$ **teaspoon powdered.** These figures are approximate, and will vary from plant to plant. Experiment to find the flavor you like best.

Infusion

An infusion is where the plant material is placed in a teapot or cup, then boiling water is added. The mixture is allowed to steep so that the flavors are infused into the water. It is best to make an infusion just before drinking it, but you can make enough for the day and then reheat it or drink it cool. Green tea can be reused up to six times, resulting in a new and interesting taste each time.

The parts of plants used most often for infusions are leaves, flowers, stems, roots, and bark. When using dried or fresh herbs, crumble, chop, grind, or slice them to expose as much surface area as possible. This ensures that the maximum amount of the medicinal substances in the herb are drawn into the water.

Most teas require boiling water for infusion. Some Oolong and black teas brew best with near-boiling water. Green and jasmine teas, on the other hand, have a gentler, softer nature, so the flavor is best achieved with water that has been left to stand for 2–3 minutes after boiling. Herbs, such as dandelion root, can be soaked overnight, strained, then drunk the next day. When making infusions, use only filtered or bottled spring water, free of chlorine, fluoride, and other chemical additives. These chemicals affect the taste of the tea. Always cover tea while it is infusing, to keep in the heat and to prevent the loss of aromatic oils through evaporation.

To infuse 2 cups (16 fl oz/500 ml), you will need 1–2 tablespoons of tea leaves or herb. Warm both the teapot and cups. Place the herbs or tea in the teapot. Add 2 cups (16 fl oz/500 ml) boiling water, cover, and let steep for 5–10 minutes. Pour through a strainer, if necessary, into the cups.

To infuse a single cup of tea, use 1 teaspoon of dried herb or tea with 1 cup (8 fl oz/250 ml) of boiling water. Place the herb or tea in a warmed cup or small teapot. Add the boiling water, cover, and let steep for 5–10 minutes.

Unlike herbal tea, green tea should be left to steep for 1 minute only; however, some green teas from Vietnam or India, such as Darjeeling greens, will need up to 6–7 minutes. When buying Asian teas, ask for the steeping time of each tea. In the end it all comes together with practice.

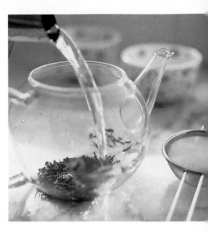

Infusion

Straining

Chinese and Japanese grocery stores sell china teapots with built-in strainers. These pots are ideal for the recipes in this book. The measured dried herb is placed in the strainer, boiling water is poured over, and then it is all left to steep. This makes it simpler to pour hot water over the leaves throughout the day to make fresh brews. This is especially good when brewing your favorite green tea. To make just one cup, you can use a cup-size strainer. Simply place the strainer in the cup, and pour boiling water over until the strainer is fully covered.

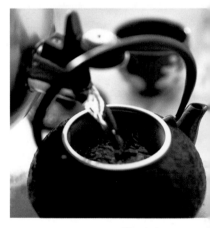

Straining

Decoction

Twigs, stems, barks, and roots can be decocted, which means simmering them to extract their flavors and medicinal constituents. The cooking times will vary depending on the type and quantity of plant used. The recipes in this book indicate the time required, but you may prefer to experiment with times to find the strength you prefer. This method does not allow for the reuse of the tea, as it extracts all the flavor and goodness during decoction.

To decoct 2 cups (16 fl oz/500 ml), you will need 2–3 tablespoons of the plant. Place it in a saucepan, add 2 cups of water, and bring to a boil over a medium-high heat. Reduce heat to medium-low, cover, and simmer for 15–20 minutes, or until reduced by one-third. Strain into a cup, then drink while hot.

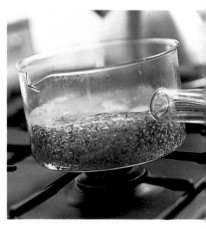

Decoction

INGREDIENTS

I f the fresh ingredient is out of season or otherwise unavailable, use the dried substitute. Generally, one teaspoon of chopped fresh herb equals ¹/₂ teaspoon of the dried herb. If the recipe calls for dried herb, you can substitute the fresh alternative. Use approximately double the amount of fresh herb. For some plants, if the flavor is mild you can use a little more than double the amount of dried herb. Note that "herb" refers to the aerial (above ground) part of the plant: the flower, leaf, and stem.

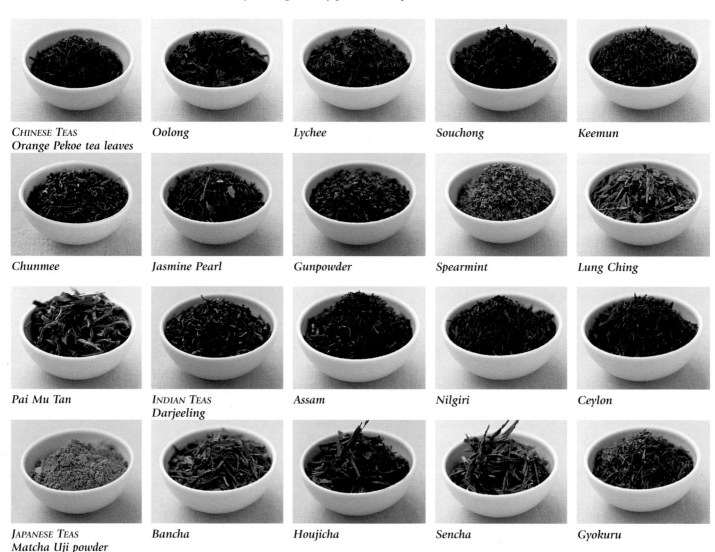

CHINESE TEAS
Orange Pekoe tea leaves

Oolong

Lychee

Souchong

Keemun

Chunmee

Jasmine Pearl

Gunpowder

Spearmint

Lung Ching

Pai Mu Tan

INDIAN TEAS
Darjeeling

Assam

Nilgiri

Ceylon

JAPANESE TEAS
Matcha Uji powder

Bancha

Houjicha

Sencha

Gyokuru

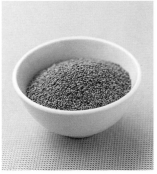

Alfalfa seeds
(Medicago sativa)

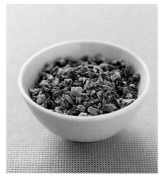

Angelica root
(Angelica archangelica)

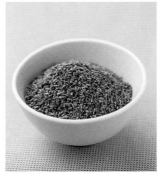

Aniseed
(Pimpinella anisum)

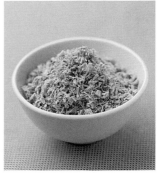

Astragalus root (dried)
(Astragalus membranaceus)

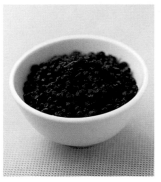

Bilberry
(Vaccinium myrtilis)

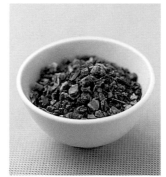

Black cohosh root
(Cimicifuga racemosa)

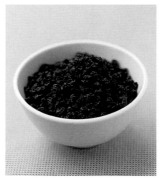

Black currants
(Ribes nigrum)

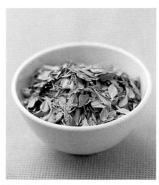

Buchu leaves
(Barosima betulina)

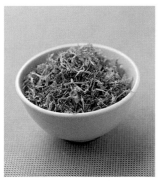

Calendula flowers (dried)
(Calendula officinalis)

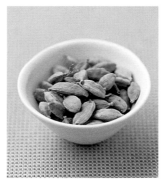

Cardamom pods
(Elattaria cardamomum)

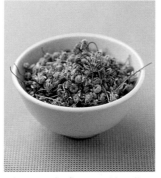

Chamomile flowers (dried)
(Matracaria recutita)

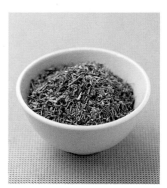

Chickweed herb
(Stellaria media)

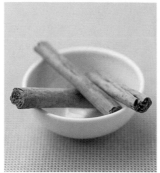

Chrysanthemum flowers (dried)
(Chrysanthemum x
morifolium)

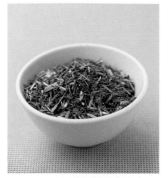

Cinnamon stick
(Cinnamomum verum)

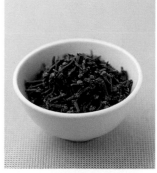

Clivers
(Galium aparine)

Cloves
(Syzygium aromaticum)

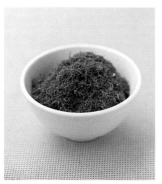

Corn silk
(Zea mays)

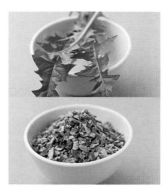

Dandelion leaf
Dandelion root (dried)
(Taraxacum radix)

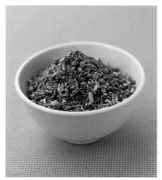

Echinacea
(Echinacea purpurea/
angustifolia)

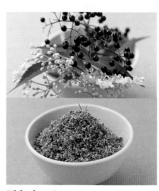

Elderberries
Elderberry flowers (dried)
(Sambucus nigra)

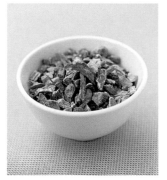

Elecampane root (dried)
(Inula helenium)

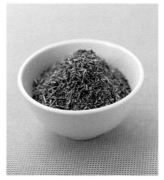

Eyebright herb
(Euphrasia officinalis)

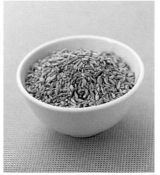

Fennel seed
(Foeniculum officinale)

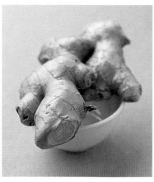

Ginger root
(Zingiber officianalis)

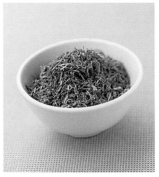
Gotu kola leaves
(Centella asciatica)

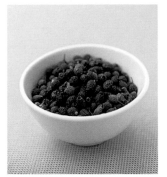
Hawthorn berries
(Crataegus spp)

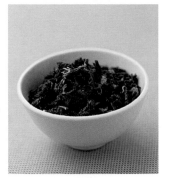
Hibiscus calyces (outer coverings of flower bud)
(Rosa seninsis)

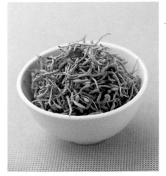
Honeysuckle flowers
(Lonicera japonica)

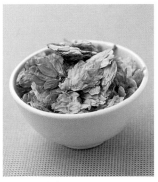
Hop strobiles
(Humulus lupulus)

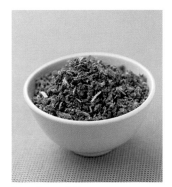
Horehound flowers
(Marribum vulgare)

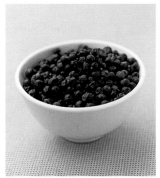
Juniper berries
(Juniperus communis)

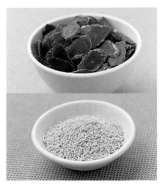
Korean ginseng
Korean ginseng (dried)
(Panax Ginseng)

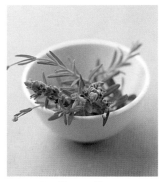
Lavender flowers/leaves
(Lavendula angustifolia)

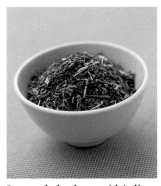
Lemon balm leaves (dried)
(Melissa officinalis)

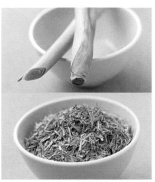
Lemongrass
Lemongrass (dried)
(Cymbogon citratus)

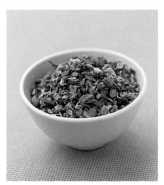
Licorice root
(Glyccyrrhiza glabra)

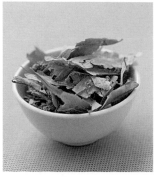

Lime blossom
(Tilia europea)

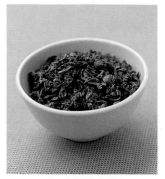

Mallow flowers/leaves
(Malva sylvestris)

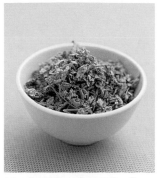

Marshmallow flower/leaf/root
(Althaea officinalis)

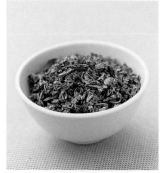

*Meadowsweet flowers and
leaves*
(Filipendula ulmaria)

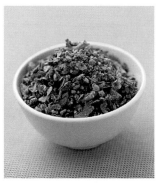

Mullein flowers/leaves/seeds
(Verbascum thapsus)

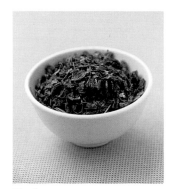

Nettle
(Urtica diocia)

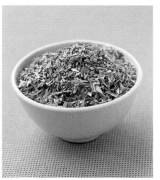

Oat straw
(Avena sativa)

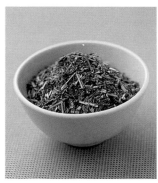

Passionflower
(Passiflora incarnata)

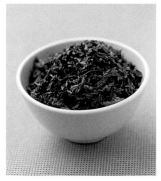

Peppermint leaves
(Mentha x piperita)

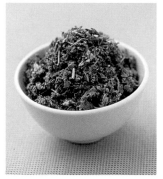

Raspberry leaf (dried)
(Rubus idaeus)

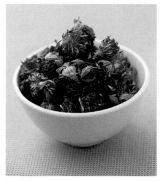

Red clover
(Trifolium pratense)

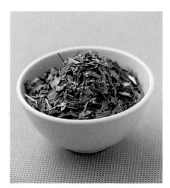

Ribwort (Plantain) leaf
(Plantago major)

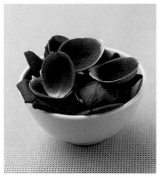

Rose petals
(Rosa spp)

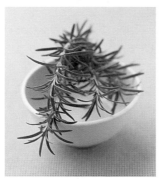

Rosemary leaves
(Rosmarinus officinalis)

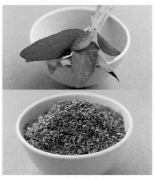

Sage
Sage (dried)
(Salvia officinalis)

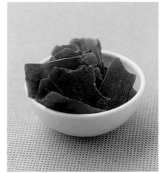

Siberian ginseng root (dried
and sliced)
(Eleutherococcus senticosus)

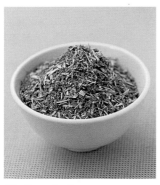

Skullcap herb
(Scutellaria lateriflora)

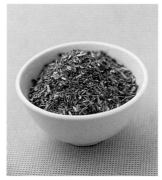

St. John's wort
(Hypericum perforatum)

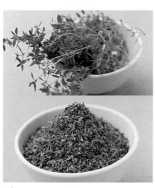

Thyme
Thyme (dried)
(Thymus vulgarus)

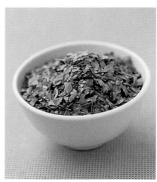

Uva ursi leaf
(Arctostophylos uva-ursi)

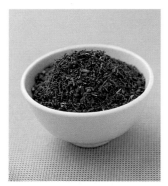

Valerian root
(Valeriana officinalis)

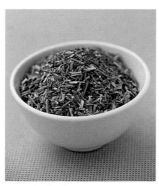

Vervain herb
(Verbena officinalis)

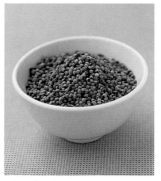

Vitex berries
(Vitex agnus-castus)

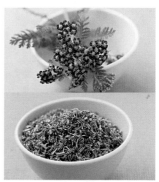

Yarrow
Yarrow (dried)
(Achellia millefolium)

23

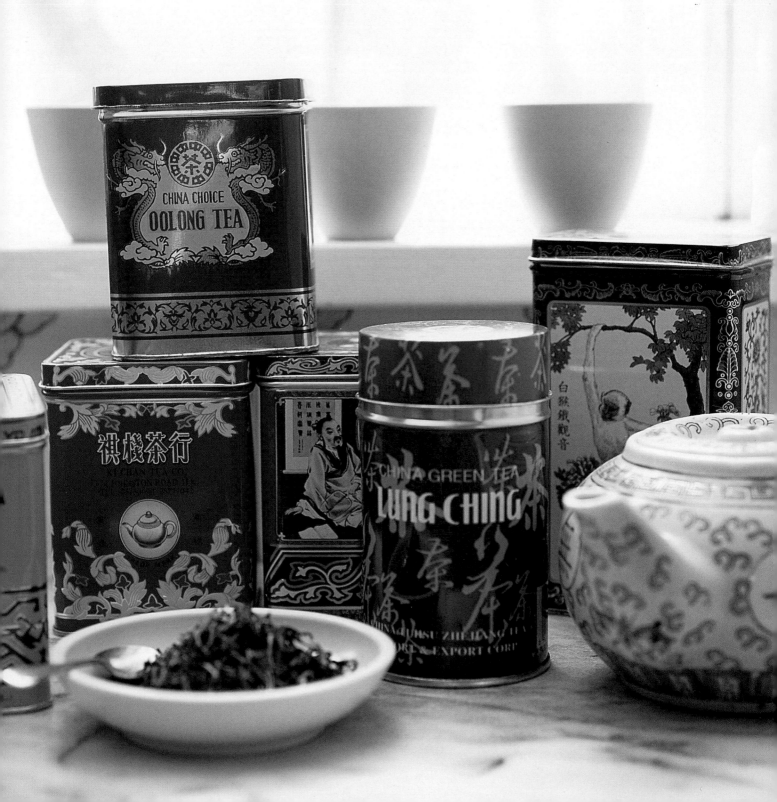

TEAS FROM CHINA

~

Orange Pekoe Tea

Orange Pekoe comes from Shanghai and has a mild, yet smoky, flavor. In reputable gardens, depending upon how the tea leaves are rolled, the whole leaf, between $1/3$–$2/3$ inch (8–15 mm) long, is known as Orange Pekoe. Tippy Golden Flowery Orange Pekoe has leaves with a golden tip. Golden Flowery Orange Pekoe has only some leaves with golden tips . Flowery Pekoe has a length of $1/5$–$1/3$ inch (5–8 mm). Other varieties include Pekoe, Pekoe Souchong, Souchong and Eshan.

Broken grades make up 95 percent of Orange Pekoe production. They are in higher demand because, due to their size, they produce the best brewing tea. Varieties include Broken Orange Pekoe and Broken Pekoe.

Eshan Pekoe Tea

This tea comes from a town called Eshan in the Yunnan province. It has a strong flavor and is often served on special occasions.

Makes 2 cups (16 fl oz/500 ml)
serves 4–5

boiling water for warming
1–2 teaspoons Eshan tea leaves
2 cups (16 fl oz/500 ml) boiling water

Fill a ceramic or glass teapot with boiling water, cover, and let stand for 1 minute to warm. Fill the teacups with boiling water and set aside to warm.

Drain the water from the teapot. Put the tea leaves in the pot and fill with the boiling water. Cover and let steep for 1 minute.

Empty the water from the cups. Pour the tea into the cups and drink it hot. You can repeat the refilling and pouring several times by boiling more water and reusing the tea leaves.

Oolong Tea

Oolong comes from Taiwan (formerly Formosa), where the climate is perfect for tea growing: the humidity is 92 percent for most of the year. The tea grows on small plantations that are not open to the public because the growers are secretive about the production.

Oolong is semi-fermented. It has the taste and color of half-green, half-black tea. Ti-Kuan-Yin, also known as The Goddess, is grown in northern Formosa and is said to rid the body of toxins and all its ills. Black Dragon is a dark, full-bodied, earthy tea, and High Mountain Oolong has a deep-green leaf that makes a fresh, revitalizing brew used medicinally for indigestion, slimming, and to lower cholesterol. Other varieties include Pu-erh and Oolong Shue Hsein.

Oolong is traditionally brewed in a Gung Fu tea set. The set consists of a small teapot and tiny cups. Only one type of tea is served in any given teapot because as the teapot ages, the flavor seeps into the clay. When the pot is older, all you need to do is add water to taste the tea.

Serving Gung Fu tea is an act of delicacy in itself. The tea is served smoothly and slowly, with grace and elegance.

Far Right: Oolong Tea
Right: Gung Fu Tea

Gung Fu Tea

Makes 1 cup (8 fl oz/250 ml)
or 6–7 Gung Fu teacups

boiling water to warm
1 teaspoon Oolong tea leaves
1 cup (8 fl oz/250 ml) boiling water

Fill a ceramic or glass teapot with boiling water, cover, and let stand for 2 minutes to warm. Fill the teacups with boiling water and set aside to warm.

Drain the water from the teapot. Put the tea leaves in the pot, then rinse with boiling water and drain, retaining the tea leaves. Immediately fill the teapot with the cup of boiling water, cover, and let steep for 30 seconds to 2 minutes.

Empty the water from the cups. Strain the tea into the cups and drink. You can refill the pot with water 3–5 times. Each brew will produce a different flavor.

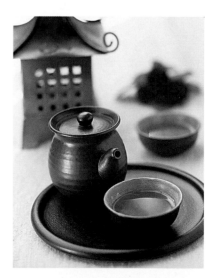

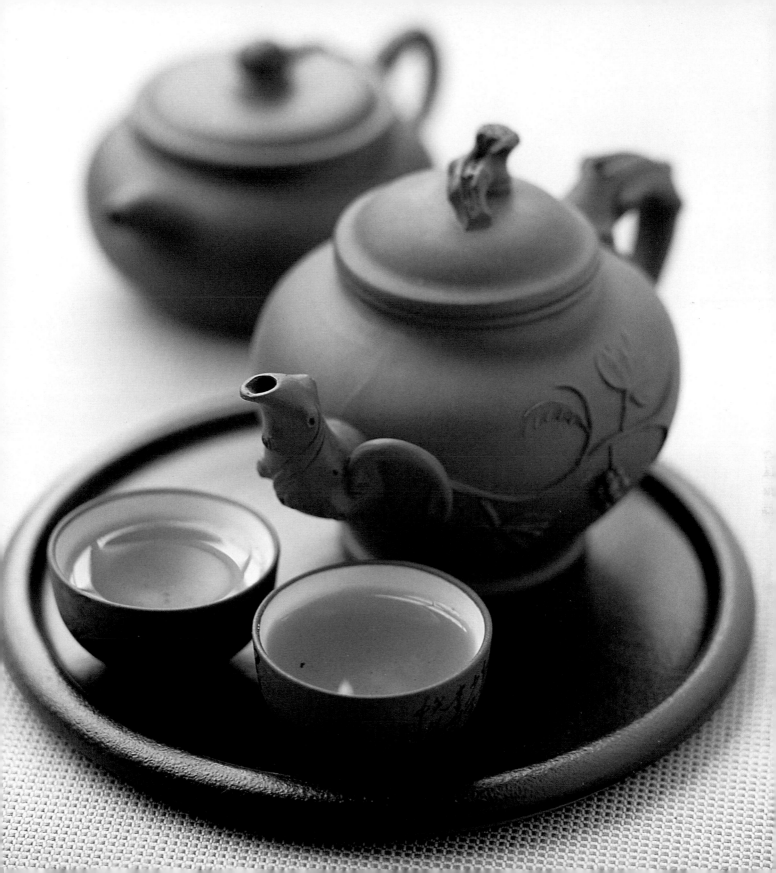

Black Lychee Tea

This exotic tea, sweetened with lychee fruit from southern China, is very popular. The leaf has a distinct fine texture and mellow taste. It is made from the finest Chinese tea leaves, cured in rooms filled with steaming lychees. This creates a sensational taste: heavy-bodied, sweet, and slightly fruity. It is excellent served on hot, steamy days as an iced tea.

Makes 2 cups (16 fl oz/500 ml)
or 4–5 Chinese teacups

2 teaspoons lychee tea leaves
2 cups (16 fl oz/500 ml) boiling water

Put the lychee tea leaves in a warmed ceramic or glass teapot. Add boiling water, cover and let steep for 2 minutes. Strain into cups and drink hot. More boiling water can be added to the remaining tea leaves to make 1 or 2 more infusions.

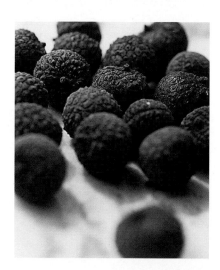

Souchong Tea

Souchong is a whole-leaf black tea made from dark leaves that are large and thick. Souchong was originally grown in the Fujian province and was known by the Chinese as Tarry Souchong. Its special characteristics are due to the soil in which it is grown.

Taiwan (formerly Formosa) produces Lapsong Souchong, which is loved for the smoky flavor developed during the curing process. The leaves are pan-fired over aromatic open fires of pine. Lapsong Souchong means "the largest leaf." The taste is mildly spicy, heavy-bodied, and rich, with a smoky flavor. The leaves are grown high in the Wu Yi Mountains, which are full of heavy mist and dense pine forests. This honey-colored tea enhances the appetite and stimulates digestion.

Souchong goes perfectly with savory and spicy foods, such as cheese and olives.

Makes 2 cups (16 fl oz/500 ml)
or 4–5 Chinese teacups

2 teaspoons Souchong tea leaves
2 cups (16 fl oz/500 ml) boiling water

Put the tea leaves in a warmed ceramic or glass teapot. Add the boiling water, cover, and let steep for 1 minute. Strain into Chinese teacups and drink hot.

Left: Lychees

Keemun Tea

This is a mild black tea that grows in aromatic orchards in the Anhui and Jiangxi provinces. It is famous for the bright-red tea it produces. The mild, sweet infusion it brews makes it a pleasant tea to have almost anytime. Due to its mild, sweet taste, Keemun tea is often used in China as a base for other scented teas. It is rich in minerals, which give it a unique color, flavor, and aroma. Keemun tea can be drunk to relieve fever and as a preventative to cancer.

Not many people get to see the finest tea plantations in China, known as the "sacred gardens." They remain a secret even from the Chinese themselves. A few estates are believed to be guarded by security dogs both day and night. High-quality standard teas, such as Imperial Yunnan from Southern China and Imperial Keemun from the Anhui Mountains, are designed for export. Keemun Finest, exported from the Jiangxi province, has a tiny, delicate leaf that produces a tea with a mildly nutty flavor.

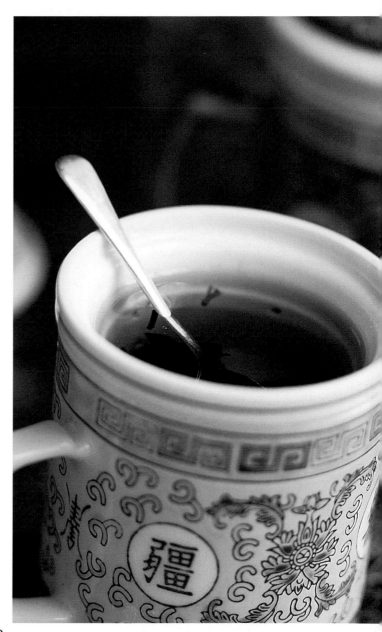

Makes 2 cups (16 fl oz/500 ml)
or 4–5 Chinese tea cups

2 teaspoons Keemun Finest tea leaves
2 cups (16 fl oz/500 ml) boiling water

Put the tea leaves in a warmed ceramic or glass teapot. Add the boiling water, cover, and let steep for 1–2 minutes. Strain into cups and drink hot.

Right: Keemun Tea

Chunmee Tea

Chunmee is well known all over the world as Green China tea. Its Chinese name means "precious eyebrow," because of the shape of the leaf. It is grown high in the Yunnan province. The leaf is processed into a hard, slender, slightly coarse, twisted roll, about $^3/8$ inch (1 cm) in length.

Infused, Chunmee is light in color, with a distinct fruity taste similar to plum. It needs only light brewing and will make a number of tasty infusions. It has the ability to quench thirst, improve digestion, have a positive effect on eyesight, and raise spirits. It is the most produced green tea in China as well as being the most heavily exported.

Makes 2 cups (16 fl oz/500 ml)
serves 4–5 Chinese teacups

1–2 teaspoons Chunmee tea leaves
2 cups (16 fl oz/500 ml) boiling water

Put the tea leaves in a warmed ceramic or glass teapot. Add the water and let steep for 2–3 minutes. Strain into Chinese teacups and drink hot.

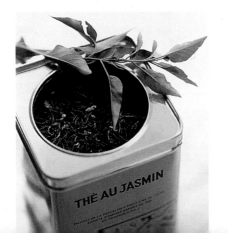

Jasmine Tea

The finest jasmine teas comes from China. Freshly cut blossoms of jasmine are added to green tea to give it a distinct and glorious aroma. This can happen only at night, when the jasmine flower opens. The flowers and buds are placed over the tea on bamboo trays and removed in the morning. Fresh buds and flowers are added the following night. This process is repeated up to ten times, until the scent is embedded in the tea. Most flowers and petals are removed after the scenting process, but sometimes they are retained, as in Jasmine Flower and Jasmine Pearl.

Jasmine Pearl tea contains the whole blossom or bud. It is fragrant and strong, and is scented by the tender jasmine bud. The tea leaves and buds are rolled into pearl-like balls that open on steeping.

Makes 2 cups (16 fl oz/500 ml)
or 4–5 Chinese teacups

2 cups (16 fl oz/500 ml) boiling water
2 teaspoons Jasmine Pearl tea leaves

Allow the boiling water to cool slightly. Put the tea leaves in a warmed ceramic or glass teapot. Add the water, cover, and let steep for 30–60 seconds. Pour into teacups and drink hot.

Right: Jasmine Tea

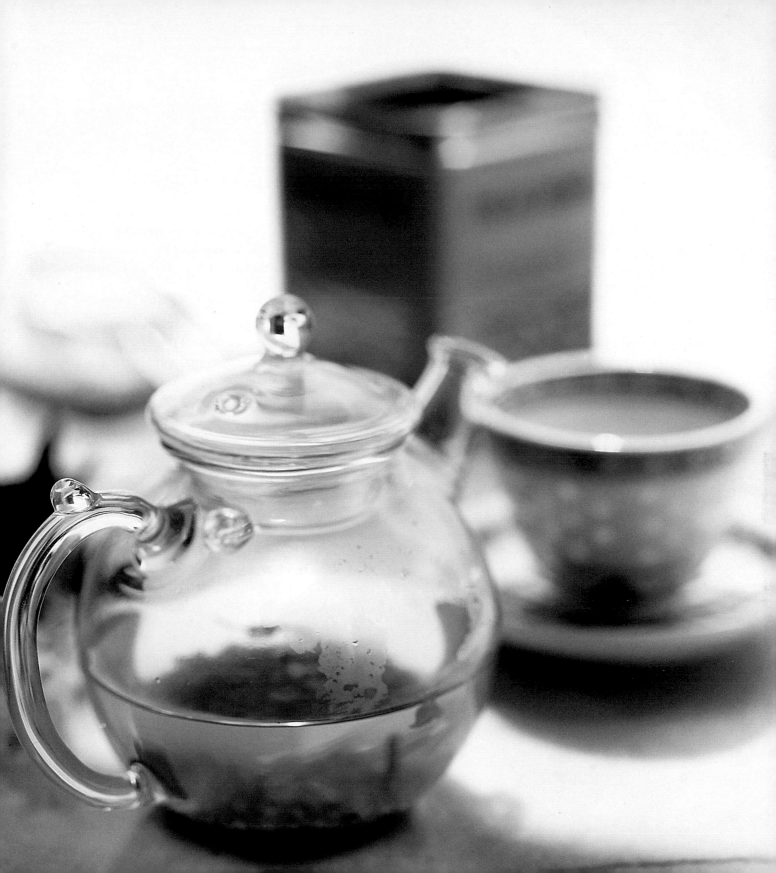

Gunpowder Tea

This is a popular green tea in China. Gunpowder leaves are rolled into small balls, up to $1/8$ inch (3 mm) wide, and are mixed with the finest mint teas from Africa and the Near East. The tiny balls of green tea explode in hot water and sink, releasing a yellow–green infusion that is very refreshing with mint. Gunpowder leaves on their own taste slightly bitter, strong, astringent, and smoky.

Different types of Gunpowder tea include Gunpowder (Xiao Qiu), a leaf that makes a dark-green infusion with a strong, long-lasting taste, and Gunpowder Pinhead Temple of Heaven, a tiny premium Gunpowder grade of leaf that can be brewed in many infusions.

Gunpowder and Spearmint tea is commonly drunk in Morocco as a sweet digestive. It has a clean, refreshing aftertaste.

Makes 2 cups (16 fl oz/500 ml)
or 4–5 Chinese teacups

1–2 teaspoons Gunpowder tea leaves
1–2 teaspoons dried spearmint tea leaves
2 cups (16 fl oz/500 ml) boiling water
honey to taste (optional)

Put the tea leaves in a warmed ceramic or glass teapot. Add the boiling water, cover, and let steep for 1–3 minutes. Stir in honey to sweeten, if desired.

Lung Ching Tea

The Zhejiang province is famous for this outstanding tea. Its name means "Dragon's Well." Lung Ching is one of the world's finest, rarest, and most expensive green teas. It can only be bought through a special agreement with the right authorities.

Lung Ching makes a jade-colored infusion with a subtle aroma and charming flavor. It is known to be stimulating and good for keeping the mind alert and clear on late nights. Lung Ching is considered a prestigious and special gift; it is sometimes given to a bride and groom on their wedding day (usually one pack for each).

Makes 2 cups (16 fl oz/500 ml)
or 4–5 Chinese teacups

2 teaspoons Lung Ching tea leaves
2 cups (16 fl oz/500 ml) boiling water

Put the tea in a warmed ceramic or glass teapot. Add the water, cover, and let steep for 30 seconds– 2 minutes. Strain, then drink hot.

Right: Gunpowder Tea

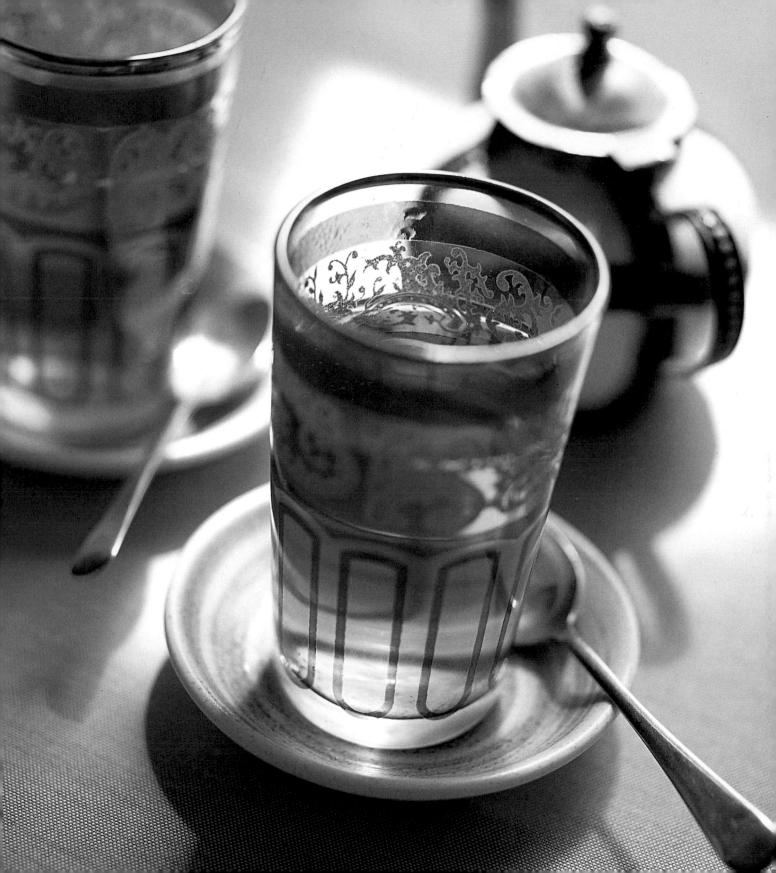

White Chinese Tea

White Chinese tea, also known as Mutant White, White Peony tea, and Pai Mu Tan, is one of the rarest teas. It is also expensive. It is produced in the Fujian province, and is only harvested on a few days of the year. Studies performed in America show that white tea may be more potent than green tea when it comes to treating cancer, particularly colon cancer. White teas are fluffy and light. When brewing a white tea, you will need to add more tea leaves than for black or green teas. The liquor it provides is pale and golden in color, mellow in taste.

Mutant White or White Peony tea is made from Dai Bai, or Big White tea leaves, and can be mixed with White Peony buds. The buds have a silver tip and are covered in down. They look beautiful as they stand upright in the teapot, producing a pale orange–yellow infusion.

Makes 2 cups (16 fl oz/500 ml)
or 4–5 Chinese teacups

4 teaspoons White Peony tea leaves
2 cups (16 fl oz/500 ml) boiling water

Put the tea leaves in a warmed ceramic or glass teapot. Add the water, cover, and let steep for 2 minutes. Strain, then drink hot.

Bac Thai Tea

Some tea connoisseurs believe Vietnam could be the birthplace of tea. The bushes that grow in its valleys are small-leafed and sweet. Bac Thai is a common tea in Vietnam and is sold at Asian grocery stores elsewhere. It is favored in hot and humid areas because of its cooling effect on the body. The tea is yellow when steeped and suitable to drink all day long on hot summer days. Bac Thai is a smooth and delightful tea.

Makes 2 cups (16 fl oz/500 ml)
or 4–5 Chinese teacups

1–2 teaspoons Bac Thai tea leaves
2 cups (16 fl oz/500 ml) boiling water

Put the tea in a warmed ceramic or glass teapot. Add water, cover, and let steep for 2–3 minutes. Strain, then drink hot.

Right: White Chinese Tea

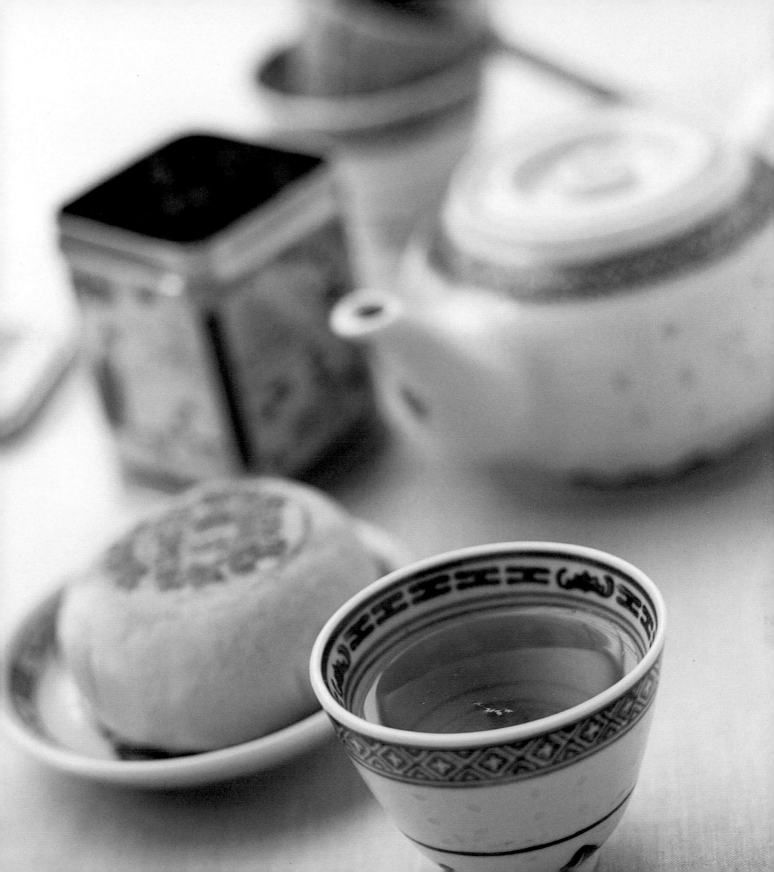

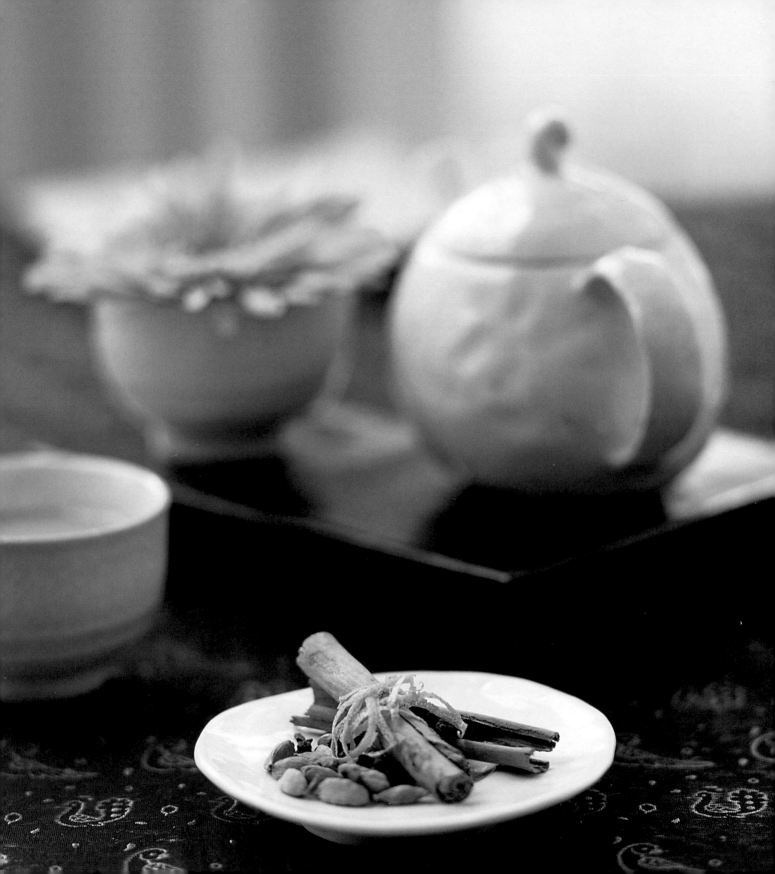

TEAS FROM INDIA

~

Darjeeling Tea

The Darjeeling region of India borders Nepal. At dawn, Himalayn women set off to pick the leaves of this tea variety that is considered the champagne of teas. The precious tea leaves are grown at altitudes of 6500 feet (1,970 meters). The plantations can produce 15,000 tons of tea a year, which is harvested according to traditional methods. Compared with other teas, Darjeeling is delicate, soft, and tender. Its popularity stems from its aromatic flavor and astringency.

Makes 2 cups (16 fl oz/500 ml)
serves 2–3

2 teaspoons black or green Darjeeling tea leaves
2 cups (16 fl oz/500 ml) boiling water

Put the tea leaves in a warmed ceramic or glass teapot. Add the water, cover, and let steep for 3–5 minutes for black tea, or 30–60 seconds for green tea.

Spicy Himalayan Tea

This hot and spicy tea goes well with sweets after dinner. It is known in India as Garam Himalaya chai.

Makes 4 cups (32 fl oz/1 L)
serves 5–6

1 bay leaf
1/2 tablespoon fennel seeds or aniseed
3 tablespoons packed brown sugar or honey
3 cardamom pods
6 cloves
1 cinnamon stick
1/4 teaspoon black peppercorns
1 teaspoon peeled and grated fresh ginger
3 1/2 cups (28 fl oz/875 ml) water
2 tablespoons Darjeeling tea leaves
1/2 cup (4 fl oz/125 ml) milk

Combine all the ingredients except the tea leaves and milk in a saucepan. Bring to a boil over high heat. Reduce heat to low, cover, and simmer for 20 minutes. Add the tea leaves, remove from heat, and let steep for 10 minutes.

Add the milk and brint to a boil over medium heat. Strain, then drink hot.

Left: Cardamom pods and cinnamon sticks

Assam Tea

The Assam Valley is 75 miles (120 km) east of Darjeeling, on the Chinese, Burmese, and Bangladesh borders. The valley was once dense jungle, but it was cleared by the English in the early 1800s. This is one of the wettest regions in the world. Every year, monsoons cause the river banks to burst, flooding the region. There are two hundred tea plantations in Assam, which yield a third of all the tea produced in India.

Only the very best leaves are plucked—the terminal bud, when it is covered in white down, and the two leaves below it—for Assam tea. (It is said that only the slender fingers of a woman can accomplish successful high-grade plucking.) The Assam tea bush, *Thea assamica*, is similar to the Chinese tea plant. The black teas of the region are grown for intensity, and are strong, flavorful teas. Only a few are grown for green tea, but the green teas produced here develop a taste that is piquant and preferred by the new green tea drinker.

Makes 1 cup (8 fl oz/250 ml)
serves 1

¹/₂–1 teaspoon Assam tea leaves
1 cup (8 fl oz/250 ml) boiling water
milk and sugar or honey, if desired

Place the tea leaves in a warmed small ceramic or glass teapot or cup. Add water and let steep for 1–2 minutes. Strain into a cup, add milk and sweetener, if desired. Drink hot.

Assam Cardamom Tea

Cardamom pods add a special touch to Assam tea. Cardamom is used in many foods to flavor and add a bit of an edge. This tasty tea is refreshing and cooling to drink.

Makes 4 cups (32 fl oz/1 L)
serves 5–6

3¹/₂ cups (28 fl oz/875 ml) water
6 green cardamom pods
1 tablespoon Assam tea leaves
¹/₂ cup (4 fl oz/125 ml) milk
¹/₄ cup (2 oz/60 g) packed brown sugar or honey

Put the water in a saucepan and bring to a boil over medium heat. Add the cardamom, cover, and boil for 3–5 minutes. Remove from heat, cover, and let steep for 5 minutes. Add the tea leaves, bring to a boil and boil for 3 minutes. Add the milk and sweetener. Strain and drink piping hot.

Right: Assam Tea

38

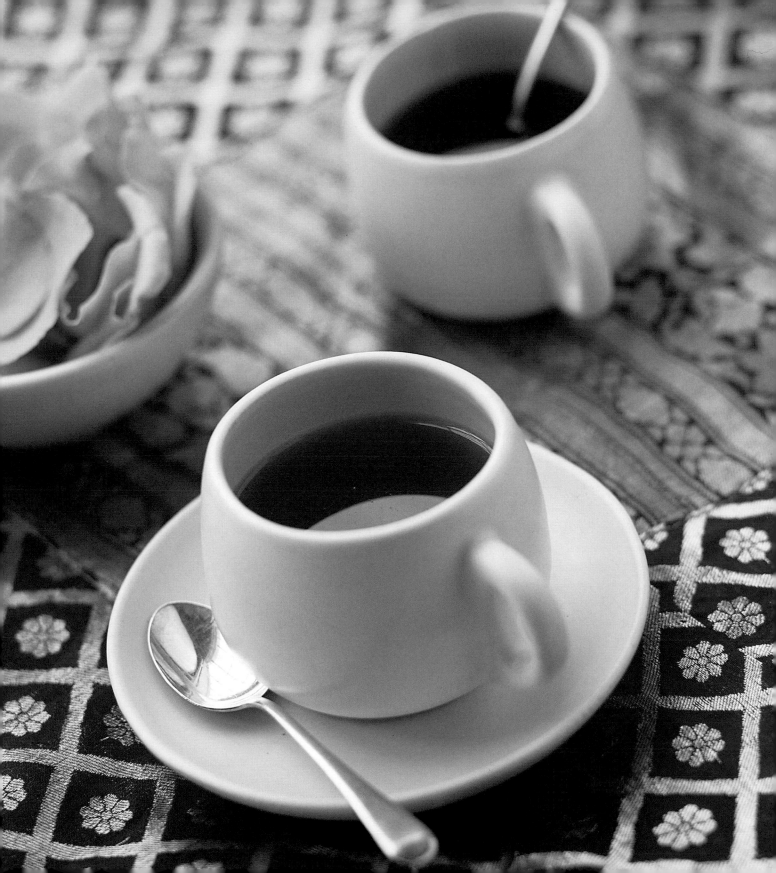

Nilgiri Tea

Unlike teas from Assam and Darjeeling, Nilgiri grows year- round. It is known locally as the fragrant tea and is ideal for mixing with other varieties. Its intense and aromatic flavor makes excellent exotic flower or fruit blends. Nilgiri green teas are delicate and can be enjoyed all day.

People living in the cooler regions of India tend to enjoy spiced teas. The spices act as a circulatory stimulant, warming and nurturing the body. Indian Spiced Nilgiri tea is delightfully fragrant and is known in India as Masalewali chai.

Makes 3 cups (24 fl oz/750 ml)
serves 4–5

3¹/₂ cups (28 fl oz/875 ml) water
¹/₂ cup milk
1 tablespoon Nilgiri tea leaves
1 teaspoon peeled and grated fresh ginger
1 cinnamon stick
3 green cardamom pods
3 cloves
1 tablespoon packed brown sugar or honey

Combine the water and milk in a saucepan and bring to a boil over a medium heat. Add the spices and sweetener and boil for 5 minutes. Turn off heat, cover, and let steep for 10 minutes. Add the tea leaves, cover, and return to a boil. Reduce heat to low and simmer for 7 minutes. Strain, then drink hot.

Ceylon Tea

In the beautiful rolling hills of Sri Lanka are smaller tea plantations where tea preferred by Americans and Europeans is grown. Over 600 million pounds (272 million kg) of tea is grown here each year. The best Ceylon teas, such as Uva, Kandy, and Nuwara Eliya, come from the higher altitudes. Varieties of Ceylon tea include Ceylon Orange Pekoe, from the high district; Ceylon Cottaganga, which is organic; Dotel Oya Oop and Aislaby Pekoe, from the Uva District; Pettiagalla Op and Matale Curly Pekoe, from the Dimbula District; and Battalgalla Op and Lovers Leap Bop, from the Nuwara Eliya District.

Makes 1 cup (8 fl oz/250 ml)
serves 1

1 teaspoon Ceylon tea leaves
1 cup (8 fl oz/250 ml) boiling water
Milk or lemon, if desired

Put the tea leaves in a warmed small ceramic or glass teapot or cup. Add the water, cover, and let steep for 3–5 minutes. Strain, then drink hot with milk or lemon, if you like.

Right: Nilgiri Tea

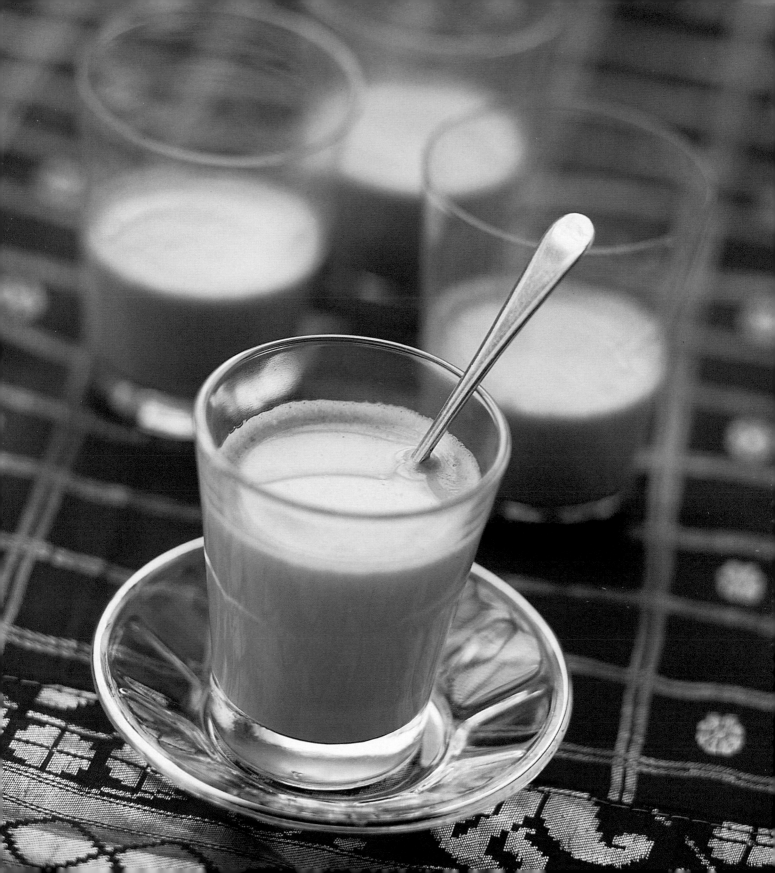

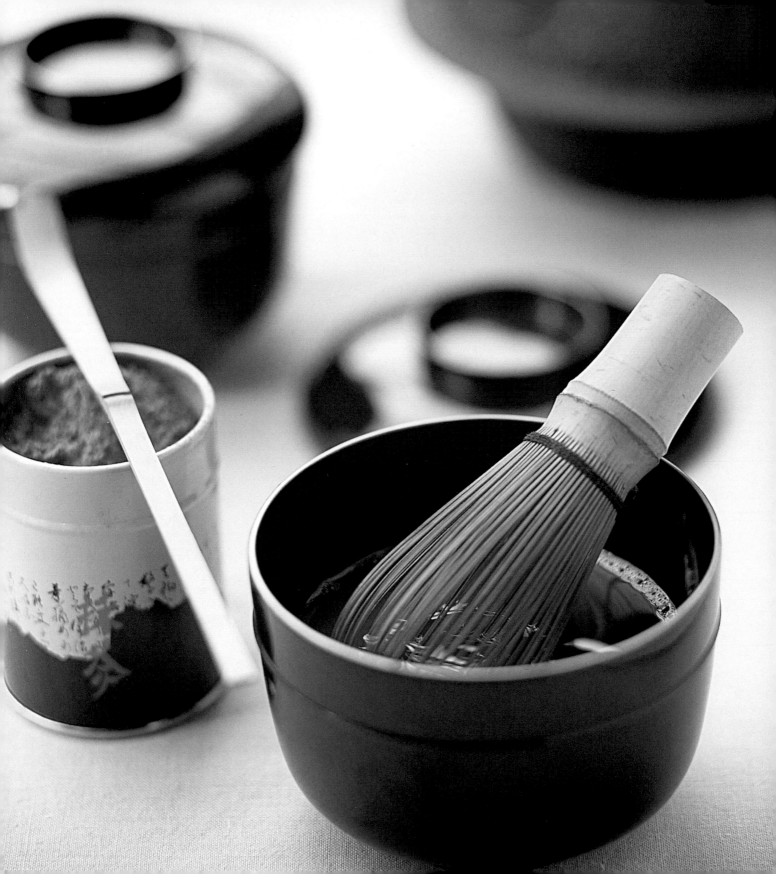

TEAS FROM JAPAN

~

Japan produces only green teas, which are grown on Mount Fuji, in Schizuoka, and on the island of Kyusu. The Japanese tea leaf is greener and brighter in color than its Chinese counterpart, as is the tea it makes. The flavor of Japanese green teas is also usually stronger than that of Chinese green teas. Japanese green tea is very high in vitamin C and is a great digestive before and after meals.

Tea Ceremonies

The Japanese have created a wonderful ritual around the drinking of tea. Japanse tea ceremonies are called *chado* or *sado*, which means "way of tea." They are also known as Cha-No-Yu, meaning "hot water tea" (Cha means "tea".)

The ceremony is a ritual created by Zen Buddhist priests over several centuries. It is founded on the appreciation of life and daily routine. The priests first practiced the ceremony during the Kamakura Period in Japan (1192–1333). After discovering that tea helped them to stay alert during meditation, the priests made it part of their daily lives. Later it became part of Zen rituals in honor of Bodhidharma, the founder of Zen Buddhism.

The tea ceremony was refined to the discipline we know today mainly by three Zen monks in the 12th, 13th and 14th centuries: Ikkyu (1394–1481), a former prince; Murata Shuko (1422–1502), Ikkyu's student; and Sen no Rikyu (1521–1591), who introduced it to the military; it then became customary for the soldiers to attend a tea ceremony before going into battle.

Sen and his followers gave the tea ceremony a style known as *wabi*, meaning "quiet, simplicity and absence of ornament." *Wabi* emphasizes four important points:

1   harmony between guests and implements;
2   respect for others present and for the utensils;
3   cleanliness (a Shinto practice that involves washing your hands and rinsing your mouth before entering the teahouse); and
4   tranquility, which is emphasized throughout the ceremony by the slow, delicate care that is applied to each article used during the ceremony.

Sen's love for the tea ceremony made it what it is today. He was a great man who introduced an art, philosophy and pleasure to drinking tea.

Chanoyu

The tea ceremony, Chanoyu, takes place in a teahouse (*cha-shitsu*), a small building detached from the rest of the house. Most teahouses are 10 feet (3 meters) square, with an alcove (*toko-no-mo*) holding a scroll. There may also be a flower arrangement or one single flower instead of the alcove. There is usually a painting, and a fireplace (*ro*) to heat the kettle on, as well as a mat (*tatami*) on the floor. The door leading into the room is low, so guests need to bow. This makes them all equal in the eyes of each other.

Guests are seated and the tea utensils are brought into the room by the host. All those present focus on the tea and its creation. This is done to create an atmosphere of relaxation, free from worry. The idea is to teach precision, poise, equanimity, kindness, sincerity, and generosity, resulting in harmony for all. The host brings in sweets, usually made from red bean paste. A sweet is offered to each guest to eat with his or her tea.

Left: Matcha Uji powder and implements for tea ceremony

Matcha Uji

The leaves used for a tea ceremony are a fine-quality green tea known as Matcha. It is made from Japan's finest tea, Gyokuru. It is dried, then ground very finely. The expensive leaves are gently stirred into hot water with refinement and elegance until a frothy consistency is reached. On some occasions, a heavier tea is brewed, called Koicha. A bowl is then gracefully placed in front of each guest, to be held with both hands and sipped. When the tea is finished and the sweets are eaten, guests can ask questions pertaining to the ceremony.

Matcha Uji means 'froth of liquid jade.' Gyokuro tea leaves are steamed and spread flat to dry. The leaves are then ground to a powder as fine as talc. This exquisite tea creates a jade-green infusion that is nourishing and full-bodied. The tea is made directly in a warmed small bowl and makes a nice accompaniment to Japanese sweets. When the tea is whisked with a dampened bamboo stick, it becomes frothy. Matcha Uji is often used to color other foods and make iced tea. The frothier the tea is, the less astringent and bitter it will be.

Note: When brewing green teas, never use a strainer or tea ball. The leaf needs to be relaxed, or loose, so it can unfold, open up, and release all its flavor. While some teas become lighter and milder with each brew, others become richer and fuller.

Makes ¹/₅ cup (1 fl oz/50 ml)
serves 1

¹/₅ cup (1 fl oz/50 ml) boiling water
¹/₂–1 teaspoon Matcha Uji powder

Let the water stand for 1–2 minutes to cool slightly. Put the tea powder in a small, warmed bowl. Add the water and use a whisk to stir briskly until frothy. Drink by taking three long sips and then pause. Repeat until the bowl is empty.

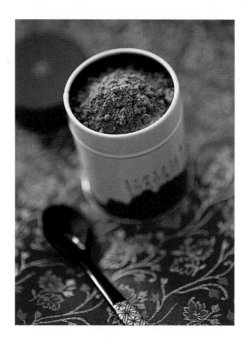

Right: Matcha Uji

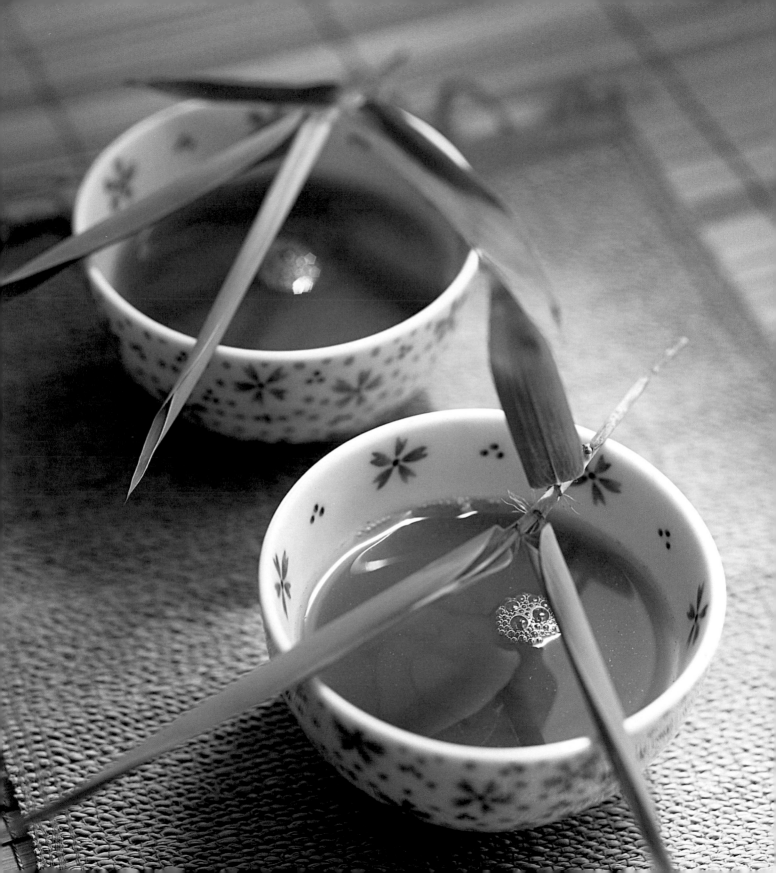

Bancha

This long, flat tea leaf makes a mild, refreshing green tea. Bancha means "late harvest." It is produced for everyday use in Japan. Considered common and rough, it is mixed with stems and other low-grade green teas. Served with meals as a digestive, Bancha is bitter and slightly astringent. It can also be served with sake.

Makes 2 cups (16 fl oz/500 ml)
or 4–5 Japanese teacups

2 cups (16 fl oz/500 ml) boiling water
2 tablespoons Bancha tea leaves

Let the water stand for 1–2 minutes to cool slightly. Put the tea leaves in a warmed teapot. Add water and let steep for 2–3 minutes. Strain, then drink hot. Pour all the tea at once so the leaves don't steep any longer. The leaves can be reinfused to make another pot of tea.

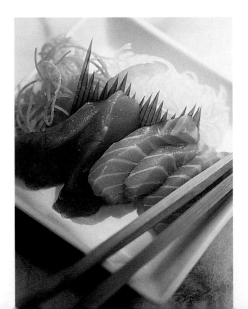

Houjicha

Houjicha was invented long ago in an attempt to improve on the taste of Bancha. Its name means "a grilled tea leaf," and it is also known as Roasted Bancha. Houjicha tea leaves are originally green before being roasted to a brown color. The tea it produces is light in flavor, reddish-brown in color, and tastes nutty. The flavor actually resembles coffee more than tea.

Houjicha is a good tea to serve with a meal, especially with savory foods such as sushi and sashimi. Its caffeine content is very low, so it can also be drunk at night. This versatile tea can be drunk hot, warm or cool, but not cold. If you are concerned with nutrients, however, you should know that the vitamins and minerals in this tea are destroyed during roasting.

Makes 2 cups (16 fl oz/500 ml)
or 4–5 Japanese teacups

2 teaspoons Houjicha tea leaves
2 cups (16 fl oz/500 ml) boiling water

Put the tea leaves in a teapot. Add the water and let steep for 2–3 minutes. Strain, then drink hot, warm, or cool.

Right: Houjicha

46

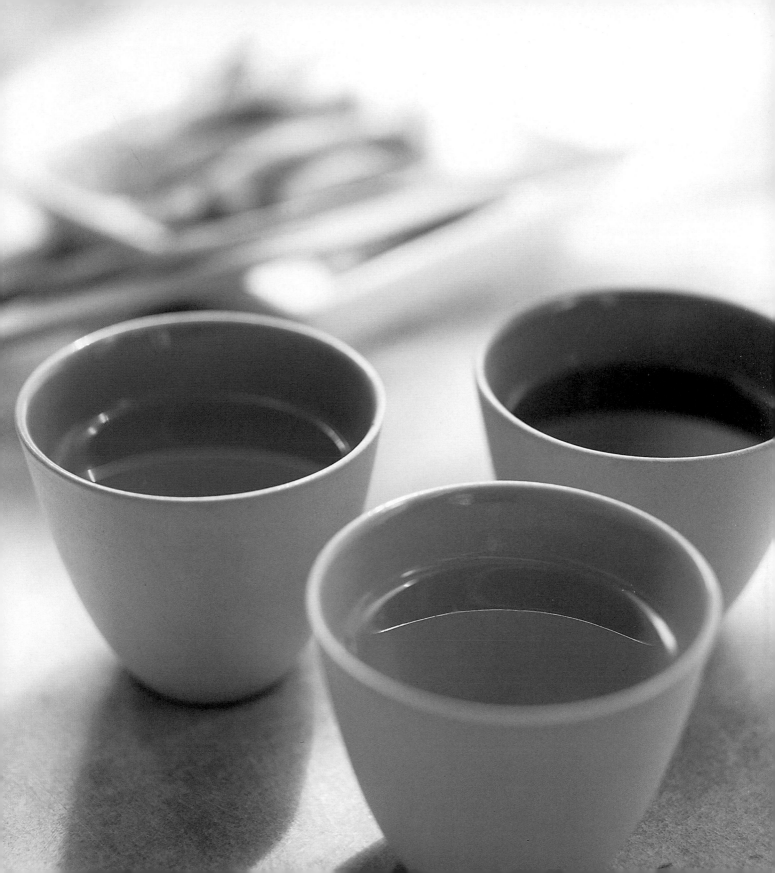

Sencha

Sencha tea uses whole, unrolled leaves. The Sencha leaf has a needlelike shape. It comes in many different grades, which are all delicious in their own right. Sencha teas are now being produced by China and Vietnam for export to Japan. Sencha Honyama stands out from the rest. It produces a fresh and flowery infusion that is perfect to enjoy on a relaxing afternoon. Sencha tea is made in a special Kyusu teapot, which has a handle that is perpendicular to the spout.

Makes 1/2 cup (4 fl oz/125 ml)
or 4–5 small Kyusu teacups

1/2 cup (4 fl oz/120 ml) boiling water
2 teaspoons Sencha tea leaves

Let the water stand for 1–2 minutes to cool slightly. Meanwhile, fill the teapot with hot water, cover, and let stand for 1 minute to warm. Drain the water. Put the tea leaves in the teapot. Add the water and let steep for 1 minute only. Strain, then drink hot. You can reinfuse this tea a couple of times.

Gyokuro Tea

This is one of Japan's finest green teas. Grown in beautifully landscaped plantations, the precious tea trees are protected in winter from frost by hot-air fans. As soon as buds appear, bamboo mats are laid over all the trees to stop most of the light getting through. This makes the leaves lower in tannin. The tea infusion is fragrant and dark-green in color, with a smooth, mellow taste.

Makes 1/2 cup (4 fl oz/125 ml)
or 4–5 Kyusu teacups

1/2 cup (4 fl oz/125 ml) boiling water
1 teaspoon Gyokuru tea leaves

Let the water stand for 1–2 minutes to cool slightly. Put the tea leaves in a warmed ceramic or glass teapot. Add the water and let steep for 1 1/2 minutes. Pour into cups immediately and drink while hot. This tea can be reinfused with slightly hotter water.

Right: Sencha

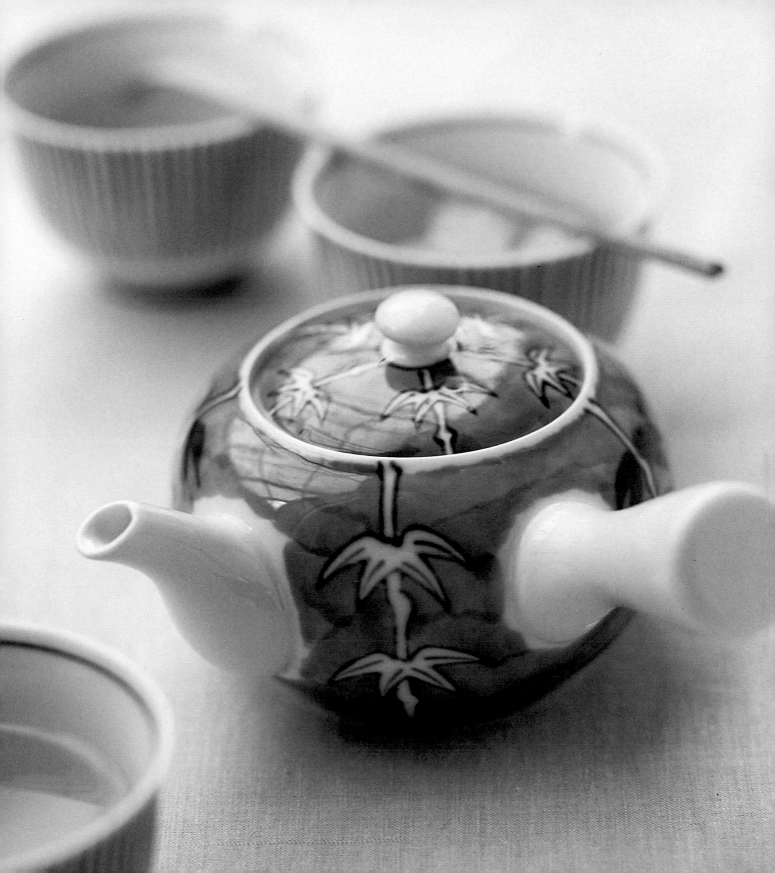

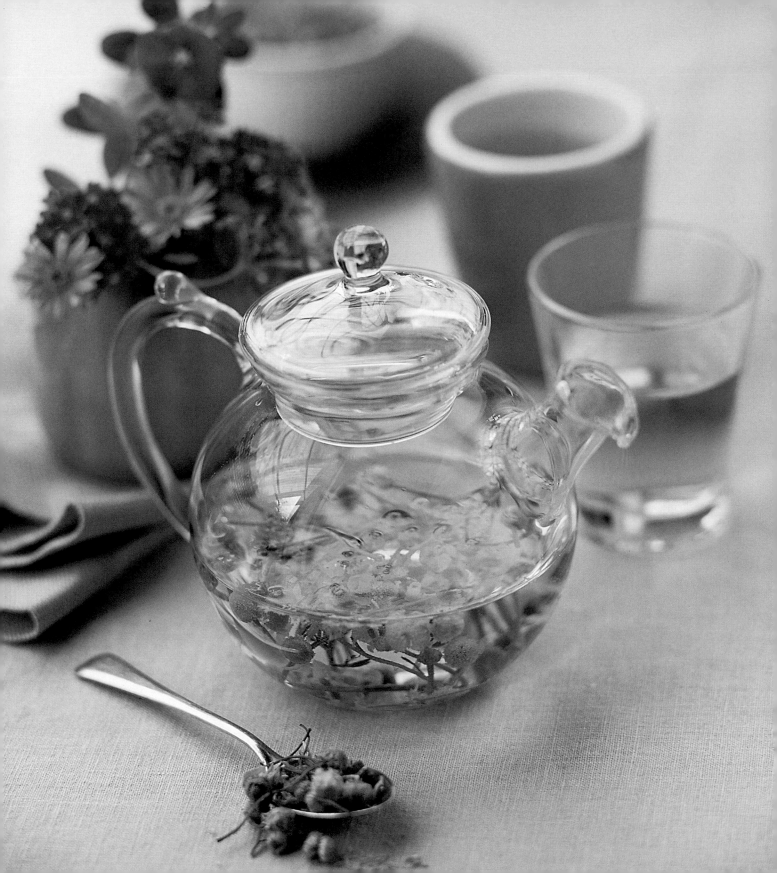

HERBAL TEAS for ENERGY

There can be a number of reasons why someone feels a lack of energy. It can be caused by constantly working for too many hours without respite, by dietary or alcohol abuse, by heavy periods for women, by underlying illnesses, or by simply not getting enough sleep. Sometimes this lack of energy can be insidious, creeping up so slowly and gradually that we don't realize it is occurring until the effects are quite dramatic.

Years of dietary abuse can result in what is called, naturopathically (i.e., referring to the terms of natural therapy), malnutrition. Although someone may be eating enough food, quite often they carry too much weight. And it's the quality of food that is eaten, not the quantity, that counts. Many people eat a large amount of fast food, which is high in fat and devoid of the good nutrients, vitamins and minerals found in fresh fruit and vegetables.

People who drink too much coffee and high-caffeine soft drinks, or eat too many chocolates, tend to feel a lack of energy due to caffeine addiction. Caffeine tends to "kick-start" the adrenal glands, which gives an initial burst of energy, but gradually tires the adrenal glands. Ongoing stress can have exactly the same effect on the adrenal glands. Over the years it can be like jump-starting a car with a dead battery. Eventually, it becomes exhausted.

We all need energy, and if it is lacking, life can be miserable. The tea recipes in this chapter are safe, gentle, and effective. However, if you find after trying them for a few weeks that your energy levels have not improved, it would be well worth seeing your health care provider for a thorough assessment.

Left: Valerian and Chamomile Tea

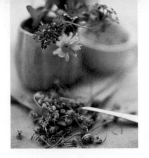

Valerian and Chamomile Tea

Energy depletion can be caused by constant stress. Valerian and chamomile will assist in helping you to relax. Neither of these herbs will make you drowsy; nor will they affect mental alertness. For the best results, drink this tea after work and again just before you go to bed. It can also be drunk at any time during the day. Note that Valerian has a strong taste and smell.

Makes 1 cup (8 fl oz/250 ml)
serves 1

¹/₂ teaspoon dried valerian root
¹/₂ teaspoon dried chamomile flowers
1 cup (8 fl oz/250 ml) boiling water
honey (optional)

Combine the valerian and chamomile in a warmed small ceramic or glass teapot or cup. Add the boiling water, cover, and let steep for 5–10 minutes. Strain, then drink while it is hot or allow it to cool first. At bedtime, you can sweeten this tea with 1 teaspoon of honey for a great nightcap.

Skullcap, Dandelion, and Cinnamon Tea

Yang and yin are important concepts in Chinese medicine. Yang tonics treat exhaustion and chronic weakness; yin solutions balance that state by providing nourishment and moisture to the internal organs. Lack of energy, feeling cold, irritability, nervousness, and a loss of sex drive are symptoms of yang deficiency. Alcohol abuse can lead to a severe yang deficiency. Cinnamon increases yang by increasing blood circulation and warming the body. This tea nourishes the liver and mind. Drink it twice a day.

Makes 1 cup (8 fl oz/250 ml)
serves 1

1 teaspoon dried dandelion root
¹/₂ teaspoon dried skullcap herb
pinch of ground cinnamon
1 cup (8 fl oz/250 ml) boiling water

Combine the dandelion, scullcap, and cinnamon in a warmed small ceramic or glass teapot or cup. Add the boiling water, cover, and let steep for 10 minutes. Pour through a strainer and drink.

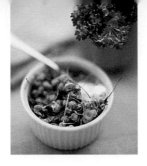

Siberian Ginseng, Nettle, and Licorice Tea

If you are always on the go, with a hectic schedule, a demanding job, and family pressures, you should make lifestyle changes to alleviate your energy-sapping stress. This tea will help pick you up in no time. You should notice the effects after a week or two. Licorice has a natural, sweet flavor that makes a pleasant-tasting tea.

Makes 2 cups (16 fl oz/500 ml)
serves 2–3

1 tablespoon dried nettle herb
1 tablespoon dried licorice root
1 tablespoon dried Siberian ginseng root
2 cups (16 fl oz/500 ml) boiling water

Combine the nettle, licorice, and Siberian ginseng in a warmed ceramic or glass teapot. Add the boiling water, cover, and let steep for 10 minutes. Strain and then drink 1 cup every 3 hours or so. If you omit the Siberian ginseng because it is not available, this tea will still be a good general pick-me-up.

Alfalfa, Nettle, and Licorice Tea

Many women lack energy just after a period. This can be caused by insufficient iron in the body. Foods rich in iron should be eaten around this time. Alfalfa, nettle, and licorice are rich in iron, and they make an excellent tea. Licorice is also known as an adaptogen by herbalists because it is a restorative and supportive tonic for the adrenal glands.

Makes 2 cups (16 fl oz/500 ml)
serves 2–3

1 tablespoon alfalfa seeds
2 teaspoons dried nettle herb
1 tablespoon dried licorice root
2 cups (16 fl oz/500 ml) boiling water

Combine the alfalfa, nettle, and licorice in a warmed ceramic or glass teapot. Add the boiling water, cover, and let steep for 10–15 minutes. Strain, then drink during the day.

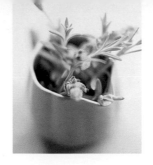

Red Clover, Hops, and Black Cohosh Tea

During menopause, women can suffer hot flushes, night sweats, and a lack of energy and interest. This tea will help the energy levels. I would also recommend a diet high in soy—tofu, miso soup, tempeh, and non-genetically modified soy milk—and foods rich in phytoestrogens, such as parsley (tabbouleh is the best source), and real licorice or licorice tea.

Makes 2 cups (16 fl oz/500 ml)
serves 2–3

2 teaspoons dried red clover
1 teaspoon dried crushed hop strobiles
1 teaspoon dried black cohosh root
2 cups (16 fl oz/500 ml) boiling water

Put the red clover, hop strobiles and black cohosh in a warmed ceramic or glass teapot. Add the boiling water, cover, and let steep for 10–15 minutes. Strain, then drink 1 cup every 3 to 4 hours. Drink one full teapot each day.

Korean Ginseng, Ginger, and Lavender Tea

Some people, as they grow older, feel they are losing their "get up and go." This tea will help put the sparkle back in the eyes, and a spring back in the step, and will help provide a zest for living once again. Korean ginseng is a pleasant-tasting herb. Ginger is hot and spicy, and is a great tonic on cooler days. Lavender is aromatic and mild, as delicate as it smells.

Makes 1 cup (8 fl oz/250 ml)
serves 1

1 teaspoon granulated Korean ginseng
1/2 teaspoon peeled and grated fresh ginger
1/2 teaspoon chopped fresh lavender flowers
1 cup (8 fl oz/250 ml) boiling water

Combine the ginseng, ginger, and lavender in a warmed small ceramic or glass teapot or cup. Add the boiling water, cover, and let steep for 5 minutes. Strain, then drink hot.

Note: Honey can be added to this tea if desired.

Calendula and Yarrow Tea

Calendula flowers (pot marigold) and yarrow have powerful healing qualities. Both help to strengthen and heal body tissues, and yarrow also acts as a tonic for blood vessels. Both the fresh flowers and the leaves of yarrow can be used. The bright colors of these herbs create a delightful color in a glass teapot.

Makes 2 cups (16 fl oz/500 ml)
serves 2–3

3 tablespoons chopped fresh calendula flowers
2 tablespoons chopped fresh yarrow herb
2 cups (16 fl oz/500 ml) boiling water

Combine the calendula and yarrow in a warmed ceramic or glass teapot. Add the boiling water, cover, and let steep for 10–15 minutes. Pour through a strainer into a cup and drink hot.

Note: 1–2 tablespoons of dried nettle herb can also be added to this tea to make it more nutritious for nursing mothers, or for anyone convalescing after an operation.

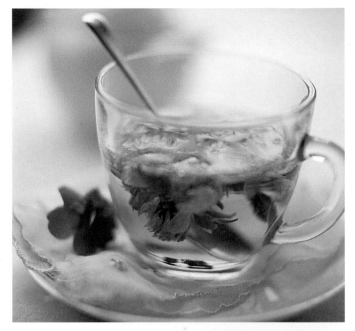

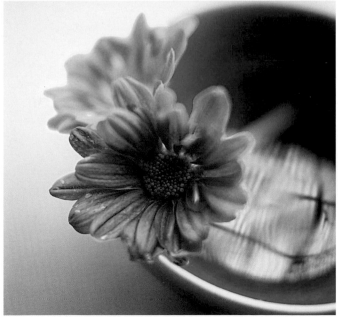

Above right: Red Clover, Hops, and Black Cohosh Tea
Right: Calendula flowers

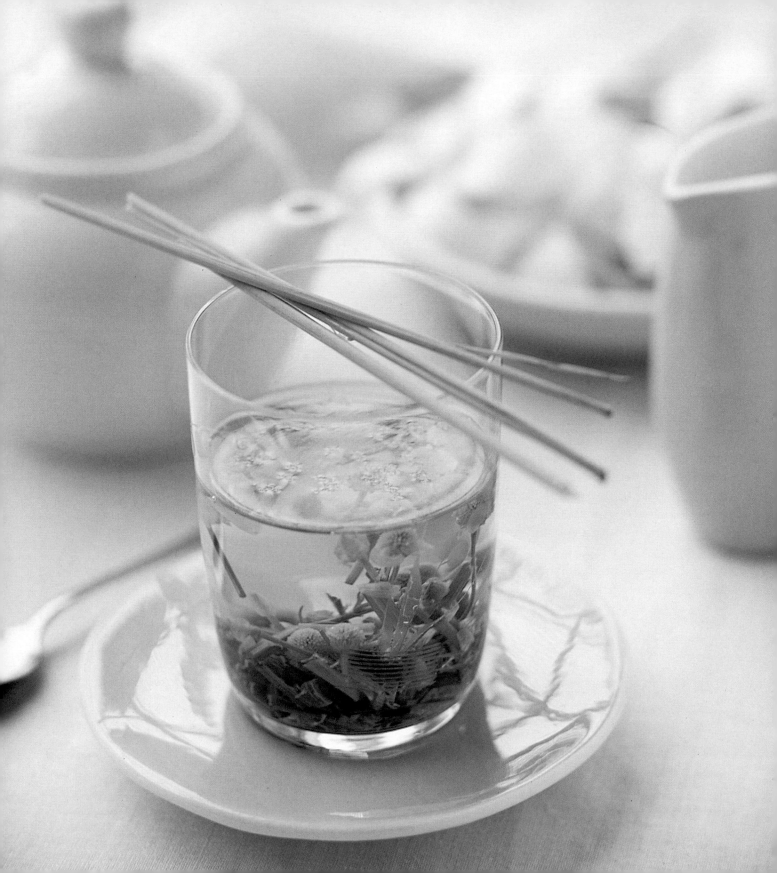

HERBAL TEAS FOR STRESS

Stress is a part of our daily life, and in most instances it is unavoidable. What can be improved is the way we deal with stress. The causes of stress can sometimes be insidious and hard to pinpoint. A constant, slowly building stress, such as an unfavorable workplace or an unhappy home situation, can bring you to a point where you can't remember when you last felt good. At other times, stress symptoms are obvious and straightforward. You can suddenly find yourself unable to cope, which can be a devastating situation.

Dealing with stress means recognizing first what the cause of the stress is, and then taking measures to address it. This can mean making lifestyle changes, dietary changes, perhaps even seeking counseling. Any positive change is worth it. Life is too short and beautiful to live it in an unhappy state of mind.

If you are stressed, take a good vitamin B-complex tablet with breakfast each day. Begin an exercise regime. It can be daily or every other day. Make sure it is something you enjoy: perhaps walking, swimming, dancing, cycling, jogging, or you might like going to the gym to do a workout.

The teas in this section help to alleviate many different types of stresses, such as those caused by grief, hormonal changes, sleepless nights, a desire to overachieve, moodiness, premenstrual tension, and low spirits. These teas will help you reap maximum benefit from any positive lifestyle changes you make, and they can help guide you onto a path of well-being.

Left: Chamomile and Lemongrass Tea

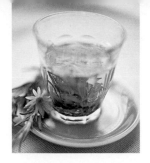

Rosemary, Skullcap, and Lavender Tea

After an unhappy event, it is normal to feel down. But if you find it hard to get on with life after some time has passed, this tea will help you let go of the blues. Rosemary is energizing, and it is an excellent stimulant that increases blood flow to the head, improves stamina, and aids concentration. Skullcap is often called the happy herb, and lavender is an effective and safe antidepressant.

Makes 2 cups (16 fl oz/500 ml)
serves 2–3

2 teaspoons chopped fresh rosemary leaves
2 teaspoons dried skullcap
2 teaspoons chopped fresh lavender flower/leaf
2 cups (16 fl oz/500 ml) boiling water

Combine the rosemary, skullcap, and lavender in a warmed ceramic or glass teapot. Add the boiling water, cover and let steep for 5–10 minutes. Strain, then drink.

Drink 3 cups of this tea each day for 1 to 2 weeks.

Chamomile and Lemon Balm Tea

This herbal tea is excellent for people who are perfectionists and find it hard to relax. If you become wound up as the day progresses and then can't unwind at the end of the day, this tea will become your best friend. I also suggest you omit caffeine from your diet.

Makes 1 cup (8 fl oz/250 ml)
serves 1

1 teaspoon dried chamomile flowers
1/2 teaspoon dried lemon balm leaves
1 cup (8 fl oz/250 ml) boiling water

Combine the chamomile and lemon balm in a warmed small ceramic or glass teapot. Add the boiling water, cover, and let steep for 5–10 minutes. Pour through a strainer into a cup and drink hot.

Drink 1 cup straight after work and then another just before bed for a restful, relaxed sleep.

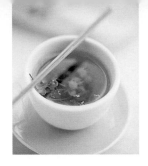

Vervain and Valerian Tea

Headaches brought on by stress can be very debilitating. Those that develop after stressful situations are known as tension headaches. These occur because the muscles in the neck and shoulder tense up, restricting blood flow to the head. Vervain is a calming restorative and antispasmodic, making it good for migraines and headaches induced by nerves. Valerian has a distinct pungent smell and works well to reduce anxiety and tension. If you drink it when you know you might develop a tension headache, you could avoid one altogether.

Makes 1 cup (8 fl oz/250 ml)
serves 1

¹/₂ teaspoon dried vervain herb
¹/₂ teaspoon dried valerian root
1 cup (8 fl oz/250 ml) boiling water

Combine the vervain and valerian in a cup. Add the boiling water, cover, and let steep for 10 minutes. Strain, then drink hot.
   Drink this tea as needed.

Caution: Avoid vervain when pregnant, as it is a uterine stimulant.

Chamomile and Lemongrass Tea

This tea should help those who have trouble sleeping. I also recommend that you remove caffeine from your diet, and avoid eating late or eating just before going to bed. Chamomile has a sedative effect without impairing any bodily functions. Lemongrass adds a pleasant citrus taste to the tea. Both are excellent digestive herbs.

Makes 1 cup (8 fl oz/250 ml)
serves 1

1 teaspoon dried chamomile flowers
1 teaspoon chopped dried lemongrass
1 cup (8 fl oz/250 ml) boiling water

Combine the chamomile and lemongrass in a wamed small ceramic or glass teapot or cup. Add the boiling water, cover, and let steep for 5–10 minutes. Strain, then drink hot.
   Drink before going to bed each night.

Note: Four drops of white chestnut, a Bach flower remedy, can also be added to this tea. This can help to calm a mind that can't "switch off".

Oat Straw, Gotu Kola, and Passionflower Tea

Under stress, the nervous system tends to give up. If you have symptoms of anxiety, hyperventilation or palpitations, herbs and supplements can help to nurture and tone the nervous system. Oat straw is a restorative nerve herb (nervine), antidepressant, and nutritive, and contains calcium, silica, and vitamins B1, B2 and E. Gotu kola is also a nervine, and is calming to the body and mind. Passionflower is the flower of the passion fruit plant, and has a sedative effect without impairing alertness; it also has a relaxing effect on the body, inducing sleep.

Makes 2 cups (16 fl oz/500 ml)
serves 2–3

2 tablespoons dried oat straw
1 tablespoon dried gotu kola leaves
1 tablespoon dried passionflower
3 cups water (24 fl oz/750 ml)

Combine the oats, gotu kola, passionflower and water in a saucepan and bring to a boil. Reduce heat to medium-low, cover, and simmer until reduced by one-third. Strain and drink. Drink 1 cup of this tea 3 times a day for as long as needed.

Caution: Avoid oats straw if you are gluten sensitive or have coeliac disease. Alternatively, after decoction allow the liquid to settle then strain the clear herbal liquid.

Vitex and Oat Straw Tea

Sometimes a period can make you extremely sensitive. If you suffer low spirits, sensations of jealousy, suspicion, or behave neurotically before a period, you could be suffering from hormone imbalance. Vitex stabilizes imbalances, starting at the pituitary level, normalizing hormonal functions. Oat Straw also helps by nourishing the nervous system.

Makes 2 cups (16 fl oz/500 ml)
serves 2–3

1 tablespoon dried vitex berries
2 tablespoons dried oat straw
3 cups water (24 fl oz/750 ml)
honey to taste (optional)

Combine the vitex, oats straw, and water in a saucepan and bring to boil. Reduce heat to medium-low, cover, and simmer until reduced by one-third. Strain, then drink. Add honey to sweeten, if desired.

Drink 1 cup of this tea the first thing each morning for 3 months.

Caution: Avoid oats straw if you are gluten sensitive or have coeliac disease. Alternatively, after decoction allow the liquid to settle then strain the clear herbal liquid.

Right: Vitex and Oat Straw Tea

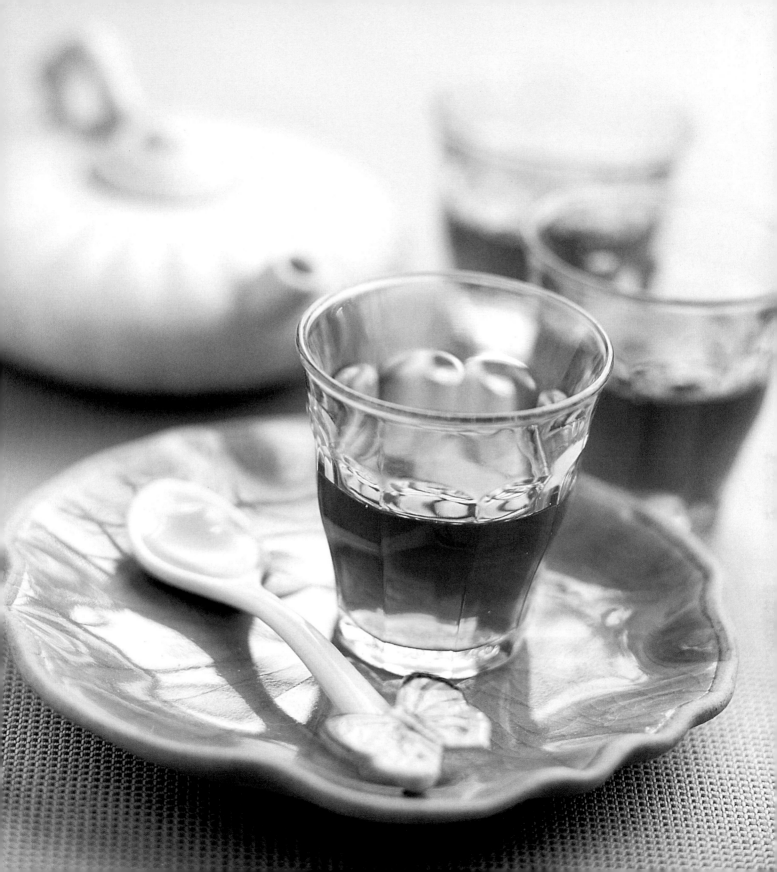

Meadowsweet, Lavender, and Dandelion Root Tea

Because of stress, you may find that you have lost your appetite and your tummy is in knots. To relax and aid your digestion, try this tea while preparing dinner. Meadowsweet is a digestive herb that relaxes and soothes the stomach. Lavender has an antistress, relaxing effect. Dandelion's mildly bitter taste encourages digestive juices to flow and enhances the appetite.

Makes 1 cup (8 fl oz/250 ml)
serves 1

¹/₂ teaspoon dried meadowsweet flowers and/or leaves
¹/₂ teaspoon dried or fresh lavender flowers and/or leaves
¹/₂ teaspoon dried dandelion root
1 cup (8 fl oz/250 ml) boiling water

Combine the meadowsweet, lavender, and dandelion in a warmed small ceramic or glass teapot or cup. Add the boiling water, cover, and let steep for 5–10 minutes. Strain and drink.

This tea is good to take before meals, and as an after-dinner digestive.

Rosemary and St. John's Wort Tea

This tea will help when you have lost interest in daily activities. Low spirits can creep up slowly, and sometimes we don't even realize it. St. John's wort has become popular recently for treating lowered activity and sadness. Rosemary is a brain stimulant that increases blood flow to the head. It also gives this tea a delightful spicy aroma.

Makes 1 cup (8 fl oz/250 ml)
serves 1

1 teaspoon chopped fresh rosemary leaves
1 teaspoon dried St. John's wort
1 cup (8 fl oz/250 ml) boiling water

Combine the rosemary and St. John's wort in a warmed small ceramic or glass teapot or cup. Add the boiling water, cover, and let steep for 5–10 minutes. Strain, then drink hot.

Drink 3 cups of this tea each day for 3–4 weeks. If low spirits do not go away, please visit your health care provider to resolve any underlying problem.

Caution: Avoid St. John's wort if you are taking blood thinning medication such as Warfarin.

Right: Rosemary and St. John's Wort Tea

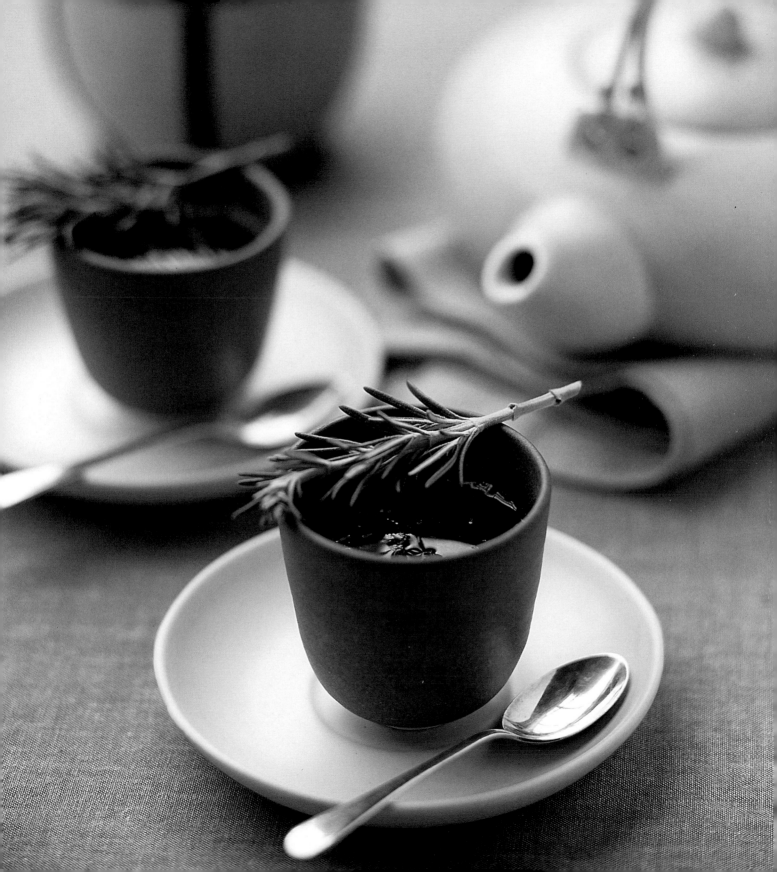

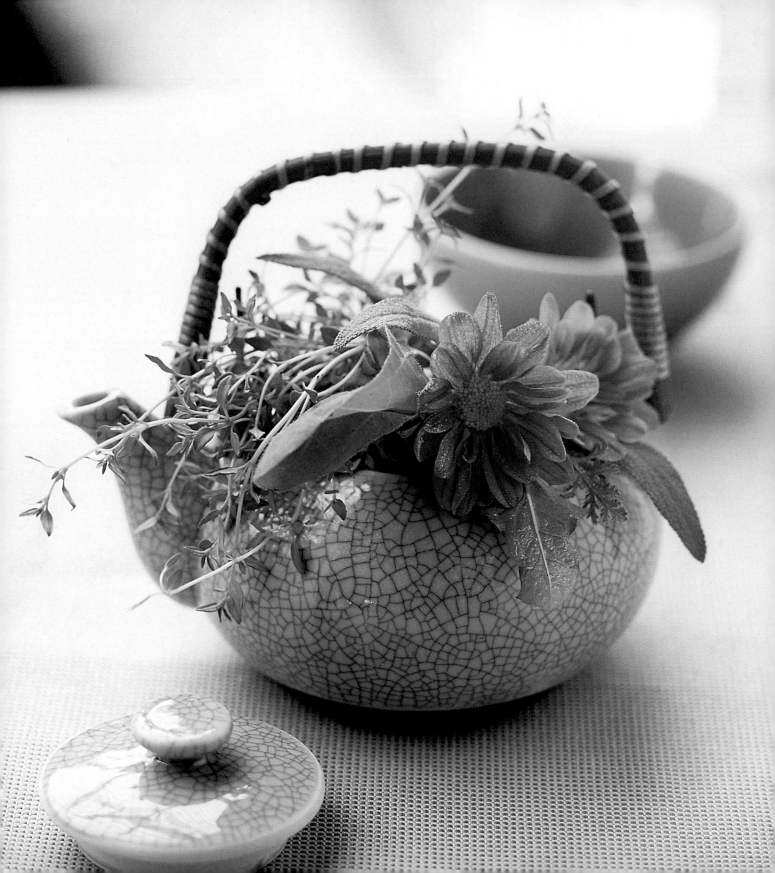

SPRINGTIME TONICS

Springtime can be the busiest time of year for herbalists. Old and new patients come in seeking tonics to combat allergies. Today, more people than ever seem to be sensitive to allergens. Asthma sufferers are especially vulnerable to allergens, and they can develop eczema or hives as well as experiencing difficulty breathing.

Classic allergy signs are itchy eyes, sneezing, a blocked nose, a heavy feeling in the sinuses, and an extremely itchy throat. There are a number of things sufferers can do to alleviate the symptoms. They can take plenty of vitamin C to reduce inflammatory reactions to allergens. They should also take magnesium, zinc, and selenium to reduce viscosity (stickiness) in the lungs. Their diet should be free of preservatives, additives, and artificial flavorings. If they suffer from constipation, this should also be addressed. They also need to wash all new clothing, towels, and sheets before use to remove formaldehyde or any other chemical treatments.

Some people may need to explore breathing therapy, especially if they breathe mostly through the mouth. They should also avoid unfermented dairy foods, such as milk, ice creams, and processed cheeses, as these products can increase mucus production in the lungs, throat, and sinuses. Fried foods should be avoided, as well as refined carbohydrates, such as white bread, and refined sugar intake should be decreased.

Herbs can be used to treat allergies very well. They mostly relieve the symptoms, but they can provide great relief. Herbs are free of side effects and do not dry up the mucous membranes; instead, they heal and tonify them, clearing the sinuses and relieving congestion. Making lifestyle changes and drinking some of the following teas may be all you need to do to improve your allergies. These teas could help make life a breeze during beautiful spring days.

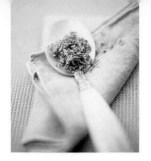

Elder and Eyebright Tea

This tea can help if you have watery, itchy, red, and very irritated eyes, and it can also help with conjunctivitis. Elder has numerous therapeutic qualities, including reducing mucus production. In the past, elder water was thought to remove freckles and whiten the skin. Elder leaves made into a poultice can be used to ease bruising and injury. The combination of eyebright and elder makes the perfect cold and influenza remedy, as eyebright acts as a tonic for the mucous membranes.

Makes 1 cup (8 fl oz/250 ml)
serves 1

1 teaspoon dried elder flowers and/or leaves
1 teaspoon dried eyebright herb
1 cup (8 fl oz/250 ml) boiling water

Combine the elder and eyebright in a warmed small ceramic or glass teapot or cup. Add the boiling water, cover, and let steep for 5 minutes. Strain, then drink hot.

Drink 3 cups of this tea hot every day to encourage sweating and to help clear a cold. It can also be cooled and used as an eyewash.

Ribwort and Eyebright Tea

Sinus sufferers feel pressure behind their eyes. This is due to congestion in the sinus cavities, which may cause headaches, a blocked nose, and dark circles under the eyes. Sinus sufferers should check with their dentist to ensure their sinus troubles are not caused by an abscessed tooth. This can lead to infection in the bone, which can be quite serious. Ribwort (plantain) is an effective decongestant that tones the mucous membranes, breaks down mucus, and clears the sinuses. Eyebright, like ribwort, is a decongestant, and has the added advantage of being an anti-inflammatory that soothes gritty, itchy eyes.

Makes 1 cup (8 fl oz/250 ml)
serves 1

1 teaspoon dried ribwort (plantain) leaves
1 teaspoon dried eyebright herb
1 cup (8 fl oz/250 ml) boiling water

Combine the ribwort and eyebright in a cup. Add the boiling water, cover, and let steep for 5–10 minutes. Strain, then drink hot.

Drink 3 to 4 cups of this tea a day for 3 to 7 days, until symptoms are relieved.

Note: If an infection is present, add 1 teaspoon dried echinacea to this mix.

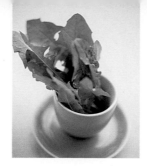

Chickweed, Calendula, and Nettle Tea

Eczema, hives, and other forms of dermatitis can appear as red, itchy rashes. Chickweed is a cooling herb, and it can soothe any angry red rash. The bright yellow-gold calendula flower is healing, anti-inflammatory, and a strong antifungal. Nettle has astringent qualities. In ancient Rome, Caesar's troops used to beat themselves with nettle to rid themselves of arthritis, aches, and pains.

Makes 2 cups (16 fl oz/500 ml)
serves 2–3

2 tablespoons chopped fresh chickweed herb
2 tablespoons chopped fresh calendula flowers
1 tablespoon dried nettle herb
2 cups (16 fl oz/500 ml) boiling water

Combine the chickweed, calendula, and nettle in a warmed ceramic or glass teapot. Add the boiling water, cover, and let steep for 10 minutes. Strain, then drink hot.

Drink 3 cups of this tea a day. You can also use a clean cloth to sponge the strained tea onto affected areas to soothe them. Chickweed tea can be added to a bath to further soothe the skin.

Echinacea, Dandelion, and Licorice Tea

If you wake up with a succession of sneezes and an unbearably itchy nose every morning during spring, try this tea. Both echinacea and licorice are antiallergic herbs, while dandelion acts as a desensitizer, strengthening the liver. Echinacea is native to America. It has long been used by Native Americans for its strong antimicrobial effect, and has now become well known all over the world.

Makes 2 cups (16 fl oz/500 ml)
serves 2–3

1 tablespoon dried echinacea root
1 tablespoon dried dandelion root
2 teaspoons ground licorice root
2 cups (16 fl oz/500 ml) boiling water

Combine the echinacea, dandelion, and licorice in a saucepan. Add the boiling water, cover, then simmer over medium-low heat until reduced by one-third, about 15 minutes. Strain, then drink hot.

Drink 1 cup of this tea a day prior to and during spring.

Caution: Avoid licorice if you suffer from high blood pressure.

Licorice Tea

Licorice is available as a chopped root or in ground form. This tea may help to minimize the severity of asthma attacks if it is drunk regularly. It is also useful if you suffer bronchial tightness in the chest. Licorice helps to break down catarrh in the respiratory system, has a pleasant flavor, and helps to prevent allergies.

Makes 2 cups (16 fl oz/500 ml)
serves 2–3

1 tablespoon dried licorice root
2 cups (16 fl oz/500 ml) boiling water

Put the licorice in a warmed ceramic or glass teapot. Add the boiling water, cover and let steep for 10 minutes. Strain and drink.
 Drink 3 cups of this tea a day if you have excess phlegm in your respiratory system.

Caution: Avoid licorice if you have high blood pressure.

Echinacea and Thyme Tea

Allergens can cause bronchial constriction. Echinacea is antiviral, antifungal, and antibacterial. It helps to build up the body's resistance to allergies. To gain the full benefit of echinacea, it needs to be decocted. Thyme is particularly good for clearing the lungs. Thyme is antimicrobial and can be refreshing for the whole body. A face cloth dipped into this hot tea and then applied directly onto the chest is very effective for chest congestion.

Makes 2 cups (16 fl oz/500 ml)
serves 2–3

1 tablespoon dried echinacea herb
1 tablespoon dried thyme leaves and/or flowers
3 cups (24 fl oz/750 ml) water

Combine the echinacea, thyme and water in a saucepan, cover, and bring to a boil. Reduce heat to medium-low and simmer, covered, for 15 minutes, or until reduced by one-third. Strain, then drink hot.
 Drink 2 cups of this tea every day for several days.

Caution: Avoid thyme during pregnancy, as it is a uterine stimulant.

Right: Echinacea and Thyme Tea

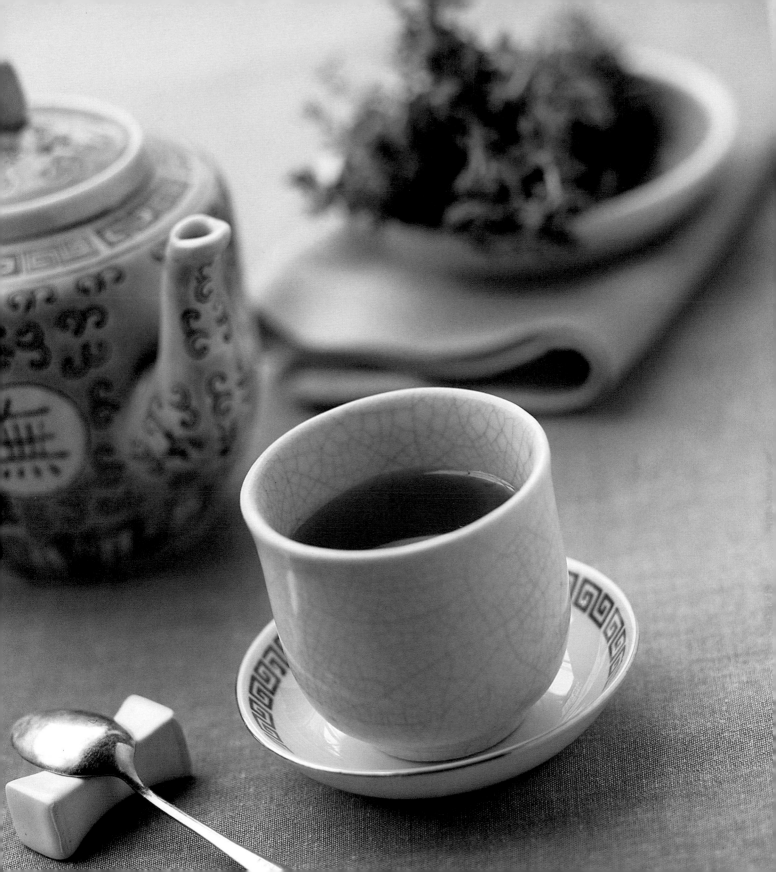

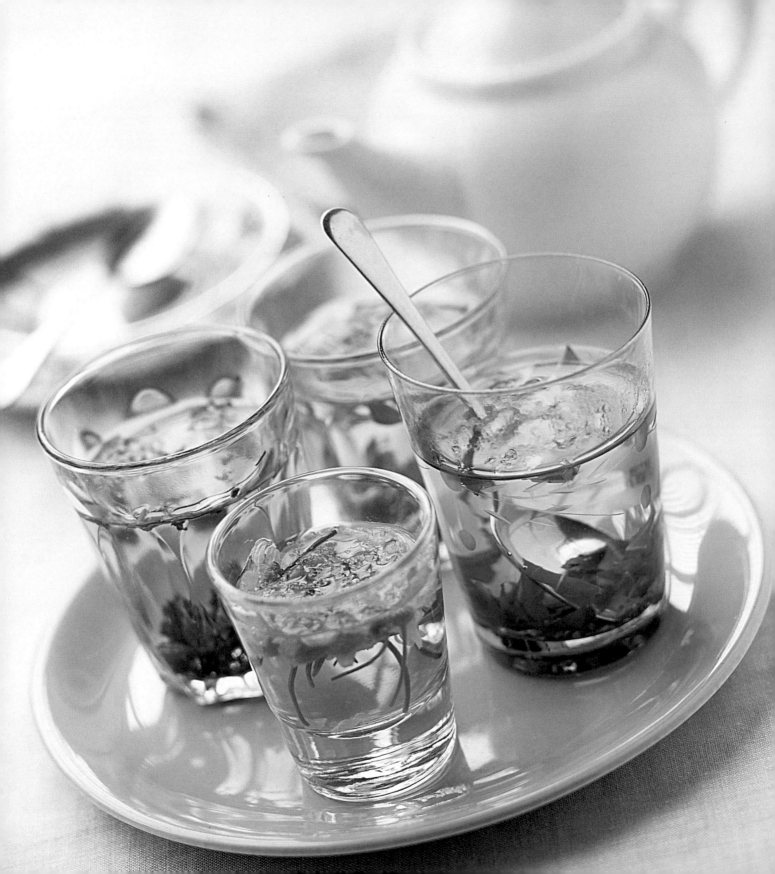

HERBAL TEAS FOR CLEANSING

Cleansing, or detoxifying, is all about improving the digestive system—your liver, kidneys, and bowel function—to provide an overall feeling of well-being. Years of dietary and lifestyle neglect can lead to sluggish digestion and bowels. This in turn can cause skin outbreaks, headaches, vagueness, loss of concentration, fatigue, and an overall sensation of feeling under par.

Many of my clients suffer from reflux, or heartburn, and other symptoms that go with indigestion: wind, burping, discomfort after meals, and so on. It is common for many people to live with this conditions for years, thinking it is normal. It is not, and in most cases it is due to low stomach acid and low digestive juices. There are a number of ways to combat this condition.

Many of us tend to forget how important drinking water can be. When thirst hits us we often reach for a coffee, soft drink, or cordial, all of which tax the kidneys. Coffee is a diuretic and can dehydrate the body—notice how dry your mouth tastes after the next coffee you have. The sugar in soft drinks and cordials are often too heavy for the kidneys to deal with effectively. A glass of warm, filtered water first thing every morning gives the kidneys a thorough flush. (Drink room-temperature water during summer.). Cleansing the kidneys in this simple and gentle way will give your body a great start to the day, every day. Add a squeeze of fresh lemon or lime for flavor, and carry a bottle with you wherever you go.

To aid your digestion, mix 1 tablespoon apple cider vinegar or the juice from a lemon quarter into a glass of warm water. Drink this before each meal. You should also eat bitter salads and bitter foods, such as green olives, with your main meal to increase the secretion of digestive enzymes. Little additions like these can make all the difference.

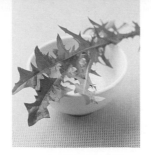

Yarrow, Dandelion, and Alfalfa Tea

Some women accumulate a few pounds of fluid just before their period. Their urine output is less, and their fingers can swell. Yarrow is a tonic for the blood vessels and acts as a gentle diuretic. Dandelion leaf is a kidney tonic that nourishes and cleanses the body by flushing the urinary system. Alfalfa is high in iron.

Makes 1 cup (8 fl oz/250 ml)
serves 1

2 teaspoons chopped fresh yarrow flowers and/or leaves
2 teaspoons chopped fresh dandelion leaves
1 teaspoon alfalfa seeds
1 cup (8 fl oz/250 ml) boiling water

Combine the yarrow, dandelion, and alfalfa in a warmed small ceramic or glass teapot or cup. Add the boiling water, cover, and let steep for 10–15 minutes. Strain and drink.
   Drink 3 cups of the tea each day around period time.

Note: The slightly bitter taste of yarrow will override the other flavors in this tea. You can add some chopped lavender flowers, if desired, to make the tea more fragrant. Lavender may also help with premenstrual tension.

Corn Silk, Buchu, Uva Ursi, and Peppermint Tea

Frequent urination, burning, and inability to completely empty your bladder are all symptoms of urinary tract infection. Cystitis, otherwise known as the honeymoon disease, is common. Most women suffering with cystitis have had several courses of antibiotics, but the infection just keeps coming back. Herbs can help clear the infection out of your system once and for all.

Makes 3 cups (24 fl oz/750 ml)
serves 3–4

4 tablespoons chopped dried corn silk
2 tablespoons chopped dried buchu leaves
2 tablespoons dried uva ursi leaves
1 tablespoon dried peppermint leaves
3 cups (24 fl oz/750 ml) boiling water

Combine the corn silk, buchu, uva ursi and peppermint in a warmed ceramic or glass teapot. Add the boiling water, cover, and let steep for 10 minutes. Pour through a strainer and drink.
   Drink 3 cups of this tea each day for 1–2 weeks.

Note: Uva ursi may cause cramping in some people. In addition to this tea, drink at least 8–12 cups (2–3 L) of filtered water daily to help flush the infection out of your system.

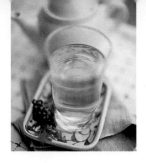

Ginger and Peppermint Tea

This tea works well for all forms of nausea, such as those caused by food poisoning, excessive alcohol intake, and travel sickness. It is also great when you are pregnant, and is very safe. Ginger is settling to the stomach and can be used on its own if the need arises. Peppermint is refreshing and cleansing to the mouth, and is an effective antispasmodic. Peppermint can also be used on its own to treat morning sickness and other forms of nausea.

Makes 1 cup (8 fl oz/250 ml)
serves 1

1 teaspoon peeled and grated fresh ginger
1/2 teaspoon dried peppermint leaves
1 cup (8 fl oz/250 ml) boiling water

Combine the ginger and peppermint in a warmed small ceramic or glass teapot or cup. Add the boiling water, cover, and let steep for 5–10 minutes. Strain, then drink hot.

   Drink this tea whenever you feel nauseous or as a preventative before traveling.

Peppermint and Yarrow Tea

One of the best ways to avoid indigestion is to eat sensibly. Start your meal with a bitter food, such as an arugula (rocket) salad, to get your digestive enzymes flowing. And never, ever overeat—frequent small meals throughout the day work best. This tea helps when you have indigestion, as the bitter taste of yarrow encourages digestion, and peppermint has a soothing, antinausea effect that eases the heavy sensation in the stomach.

Makes 1 cup (8 fl oz/250 ml)
serves 1

2 teaspoons chopped fresh yarrow leaves and/or flowers
1 teaspoon dried peppermint leaves
1 cup (8 fl oz/250 ml) boiling water

Combine the peppermint and yarrow in a warmed small ceramic or glass teapot or cup. Add the boiling water, cover, and let steep for 5–10 minutes. Strain, then drink hot.

   Drink 1 cup of this tea after a heavy meal or when you suffer with indigestion.

Dandelion Tea

The young, jagged, toothlike leaves of the dandelion plant make a delicious bitter addition to salads and are great as a kidney tonic in tea. Dandelion leaf is one of the strongest diuretics, and it is rich in potassium. Dandelion root tastes bitter. It is used to treat liver conditions, and to help with constipation and jaundice.

Makes 1 cup (8 fl oz/250 ml)
serves 1

2 teaspoons dried dandelion root, or 1 tablespoon chopped
fresh dandelion leaf
1 cup (8 fl oz/250 ml) water

Combine the dandelion root or leaf in a glass and add the water. Cover and let soak overnight. Strain and drink.
   Drink 1 to 2 cups of this tea daily.

Dandelion, Licorice, and Ginger Tea

Binge drinking is harmful to the body. If you know you are going to drink a lot of alcohol, make sure you take a vitamin B-complex tablet and 3,000 mg vitamin C pre- and post-drinking, with some food. One of the best preventatives of alcohol dehydration is drinking an equal amount of water with alcohol during the evening. This tea can help after a big night out. The bitter dandelion root will rejuvenate the liver, while the sweet-tasting licorice acts as an adaptogen for the adrenals, cleansing and nourishing the system. Ginger can settle that seedy feeling in the stomach.

Makes 2 cups (16 fl oz/500 ml)
serves 2–3

1 teaspoon dried dandelion root
1/2 teaspoon ground licorice root
1/2 teaspoon peeled and grated fresh ginger
2 cups (16 fl oz/500 ml) boiling water

Combine the dandelion, licorice and ginger in a warmed ceramic or glass teapot. Add the boiling water, cover, and let steep for 10 minutes. Pour through a strainer into a warmed cup and drink.
   Drink 1 to 2 cups of this tea on rising and then 1 cup each day for 1 week to help the body regain strength.

Right: Dandelion Tea

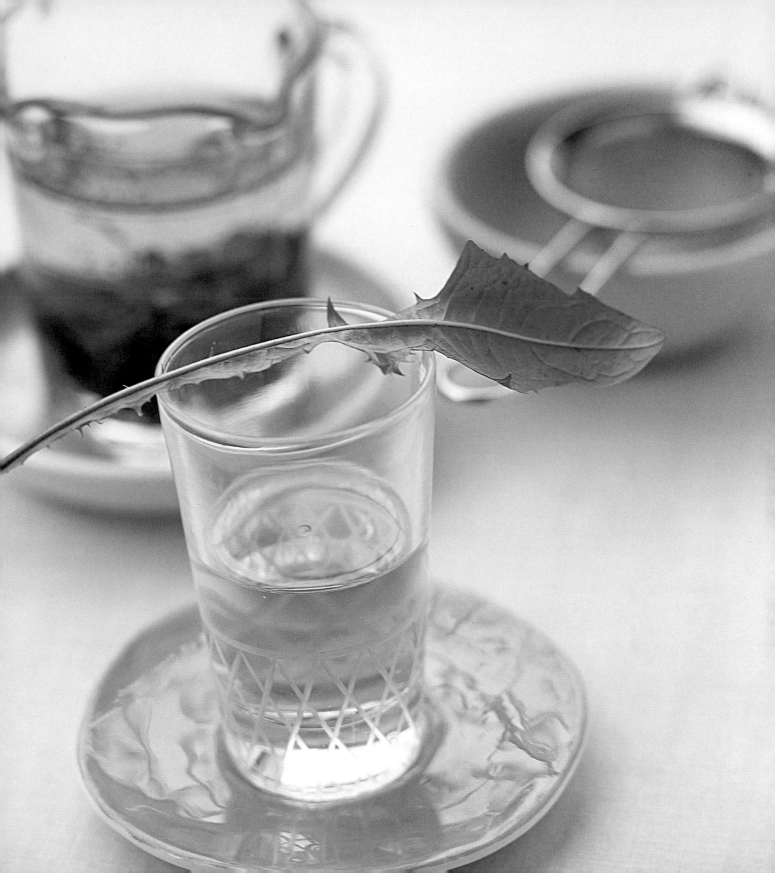

Chamomile and Aniseed Tea

This tea is gentle, safe, and delicious to drink. It can quickly soothe and quiet a frantic, colicky baby, but be sure to boil the water for 10 minutes when preparing a bottle for a baby, to ensure that you kill all the bacteria. Chamomile is antispasmodic and a relaxant. Aniseed adds a menthol-like taste to the tea and acts as a carminative by helping to reduce flatulence and cramping.

Makes 1/2 cup (4 fl oz/125 ml)
serves 1

1 teaspoon dried chamomile flowers
1/2 teaspoon aniseed, slightly crushed
1/2 cup (4 fl oz/125 ml) boiling water

Combine the chamomile and aniseed in a warmed small ceramic or glass teapot or cup. Add the boiling water, cover, and let steep for 5–10 minutes. Allow to cool to lukewarm for babies. Strain, then drink.

Caution: Honey can be added to sweeten, but do not add when preparing for babies under 2 years of age.

Nettle and Clivers Tea

This tea is nourishing and cleansing for the lymphatic system. Nettle is rich in iron and vitamin C and is supportive for the whole body. It is a great treatment for gout, allergic reactions such as hives and eczema, and for debility. Clivers is one of the best lymphatic herbs for those who suffer recurrent sore throats or persistent swollen glands, especially after glandular fever. It clears congested lymph nodes.

Makes 2 cups (16 fl oz/500 ml)
serves 2–3

2–3 tablespoons dried nettle herb
2–3 tablespoons dried clivers
2 cups (16 fl oz/500 ml) boiling water

Combine the nettle and clivers in a warmed ceramic or glass teapot. Add the boiling water, cover, and let steep for 10–15 minutes. Strain, then drink.
  Drink up to 3 cups of this tea each day.

Right: Chamomile and Aniseed Tea

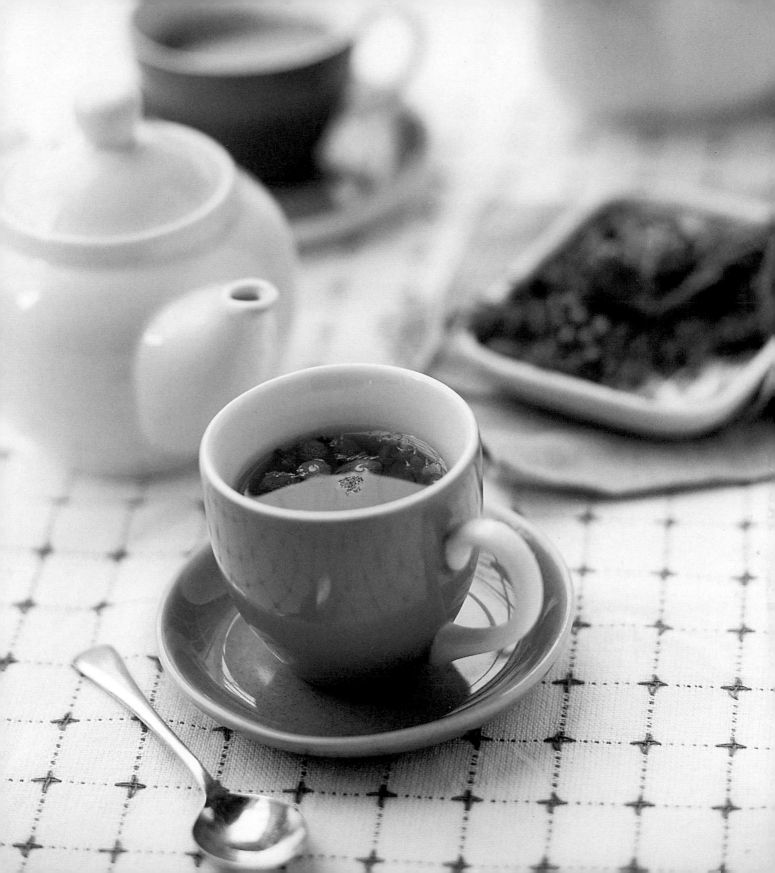

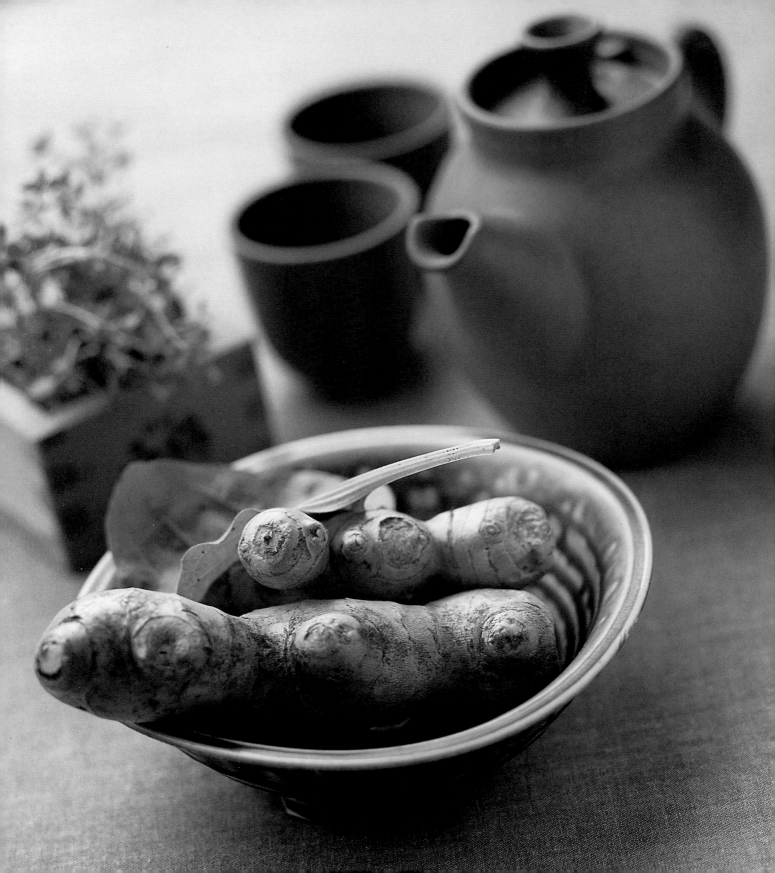

HERBAL TEAS FOR IMMUNITY

Have you noticed how often people catch a cold or the flu these days? Getting sick once in a while is normal. Naturopathically, catching a cold every few years is thought of as a good cleansing. Children get sick more often than adults, as they still need to build up resistance and strengthen their immune system. But it is thought that the heavy use of antibiotics in our society has worked against us. Many strains of microbes have become resistant to antibiotics. They have mutated (changed their form), and the antibiotics don't work as well they used to, if at all, against them. And our bodies are less resistant to these microbes, causing more illnesses.

Instead of becoming reliant on antibiotics to cure our ills, we should look for ways to prevent these common diseases. The best way to do this is to eat well-balanced, wholesome meals that are pesticide and additive free, and made with fresh ingredients. We should also make our homes and workplaces more safe by using fewer sprays, chemical cleaners, and insect repellents.

Zinc is responsible for many functions in the body; one of them is immunity. If the body is low in zinc, it can be susceptible to colds, coughs, and recurrent sore throats. Foods that are rich in zinc include oysters, seafood, pumpkin seeds (pepitas), and sunflower seeds.

The following teas are useful as preventatives and for halting an infection in its track. They include some that will soothe sore and scratchy throats, ease a cough, expel mucus, and help you sweat an illness out and make a full recovery. Keep in mind that teas are not as strong as a liquid extract that an herbalist might prescribe. If symptoms do not go away, visit your health care provider for a thorough assessment.

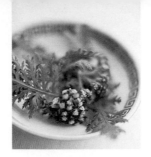

Licorice, Ginger, and Yarrow Tea

This delicious tea will create an inner warmth to help you survive cold, gloomy winter days. It is a good all-round tonic. Licorice is particularly helpful for treating upper and lower respiratory conditions and is used extensively in Chinese and Western herbal medicine. Ginger is warming and soothing to the chest and stomach. Yarrow, like ginger, acts as a diaphoretic (brings on a sweat), and is a decongestant with strong antiallergenic properties.

Makes 1 cup (8 fl oz/250 ml)
serves 1

1 tablespoon chopped fresh yarrow leaves and/or flowers
¹/₂ teaspoon ground licorice root
¹/₂ teaspoon peeled and grated fresh ginger
1 cup (8 fl oz/250 ml) boiling water

Combine the yarrow, licorice and ginger in a warmed small ceramic or glass teapot or cup. Add the boiling water, cover, and let steep for 3–5 minutes. Strain and drink.

Drink 1 cup of this tea each day approaching, and during, winter.

Cautions: Licorice should be avoided if you have high blood pressure. Yarrow should be avoided during pregnancy.

Licorice and Ginger Tea

If you feel a cold coming on, drink this tea quick! It will help to expel heat from your body, bringing on a good sweat to help your body fight the infection and cool down. Licorice is a sweet and pleasant-tasting herb. Ginger is hot and warming; the quantity might need to be adjusted to suit your taste buds. The more ginger you use the better its effect.

Makes about 3 cups (24 fl oz/750 ml)
serves 4–5

2 tablespoons ground licorice root
2 tablespoons peeled and grated fresh ginger
3 cups (24 fl oz/750 ml) boiling water

Combine the licorice and ginger in a warmed ceramic or glass teapot. Add the boiling water, cover, and let steep for 5–10 minutes. Strain, then drink piping hot.

It's important to drink this tea while it's hot, to encourage your body to sweat—this will help your body to fight the virus. Aim to drink 1 cup every 1 to 2 hours on the first day, then gradually taper off to 2 to 4 cups a day for up to 4 days, or until symptoms subside.

Caution: Avoid licorice if you have high blood pressure.

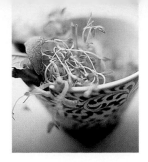

Goldenrod, Eyebright, and Ribwort Tea

This tea is for both children and adults. Goldenrod, eyebright, and ribwort (plaintain) are decongestants, tonics to the mucous membranes. For this reason, this tea is good for those who have an intolerance to dairy products. Eyebright is the first thing I think of for mucous membrane conditions. Goldenrod is antiseptic and anti-inflammatory. Ribwort is also anti-inflammatory, grows everywhere as a weed, and can be plucked out of the garden or used dry.

Makes 2 cups (16 fl oz/500 ml)
serves 2–3

1 teaspoon dried goldenrod herb
2 teaspoons dried eyebright herb
2 teaspoons dried ribwort (plantain) leaves
2 cups (16 fl oz/500 ml) boiling water

Combine the goldenrod, eyebright, and ribwort in a warmed ceramic or glass teapot. Add the boiling water, cover, and let steep for 10 minutes.

Drink 3 cups of this tea a day for a week or so.

Note: This tea can be varied by using only two of the herbs, if desired, or by adding 1 teaspoon of ground licorice root for its added effect and taste.

Caution: Avoid licorice if you have high blood pressure.

Horehound, Mullein, and Thyme Tea

A buildup of mucus in the throat and lungs can linger if not cleared promptly and effectively. Horehound has a gentle, stimulating, expectorant action on the lungs, which encourages the clearance of phlegm. This makes it good for treating bronchitis and asthma. Mullein soothes itchy and irritating coughs. Thyme is a strong antimicrobial, antispasmodic, and relaxant for the bronchi. Thyme tea on its own makes a great gargle for gum disease and sore throats.

Makes 2 cups (16 fl oz/500 ml)
serves 2–3

2 teaspoons dried horehound flowers and/or leaves
2 teaspoons dried mullein flowers and/or leaves
2 teaspoons dried thyme herb
2 cups (16 fl oz/500 ml) boiling water

Combine the horehound, mullein, and thyme in a warmed ceramic or glass teapot. Add the boiling water, cover, and let steep for 10 minutes. Strain, then drink hot.

Drink 2–3 cups a day of this tea while it is quite hot, for 5–6 days, or until your chest has cleared.

Caution: Avoid thyme during pregnancy, as it is a uterine stimulant.

Sage and Astragalus Tea

This tea is recommended for those who suffer recurrent sore throats and swollen glands. It does wonders after a bout of glandular fever, as it cleanses and clears congestion in the lymphatic system. Bacteria that thrive in an inflamed throat love sugar, because it gives them food so they can multiply, so you should also avoid all foods containing sugar and refined carbohydrates. Sage is strong in taste, antimicrobial, and makes an excellent gargle on its own. Astragalus is a sweet and warming immunostimulant herb that encourages healing and tissue regeneration.

Makes 1 cup (8 fl oz/250 ml)
serves 1

2 teaspoons crumbled dried sage leaves, or
1 tablespoon chopped fresh sage
1 teaspoon dried astragalus root
1 cup (8 fl oz/250 ml) boiling water

Combine the sage and astragalus in a warmed small ceramic or glass teapot or cup. Add the boiling water and let steep for 5 minutes. Strain and drink.

Drink 1 cup of this tea twice a day for 1 week.

Caution: Sage should be avoided if you have epilepsy.

Licorice and Echinacea Tea

A healthy liver plays an important role in managing allergies, as it helps to minimize reactions. Being aware of what you put in your body, and what you expose it to, can and will make all the difference. Licorice and echinacea both strengthen the body's defenses and help it to be less reactive to allergens. Licorice is a tonic for the liver and encourages regular bowel motions so that constipation is avoided. Echinacea is an effective immunostimulant and antimicrobial, with the fresh plant being more potent than the dried.

Makes 2 cups (16 fl oz/500 ml)
serves 2–3

1 tablespoon dried licorice root
2 tablespoons chopped fresh echinacea flowers/roots or
1 tablespoon dried echinacea root
3 cups (16 fl oz/500 ml) boiling water

Combine the licorice, echinacea, and water in a medium saucepan. Bring to a boil over high heat. Reduce heat to medium-low, cover, then simmer for 15 minutes, or until reduced by one-third. Strain, then drink hot.

Drink 1 to 2 cups of this tea a day as a preventative, or 3 cups a day during illness.

Caution: Licorice should be avoided if you have high blood pressure.

Right: Sage and Astragalus Tea

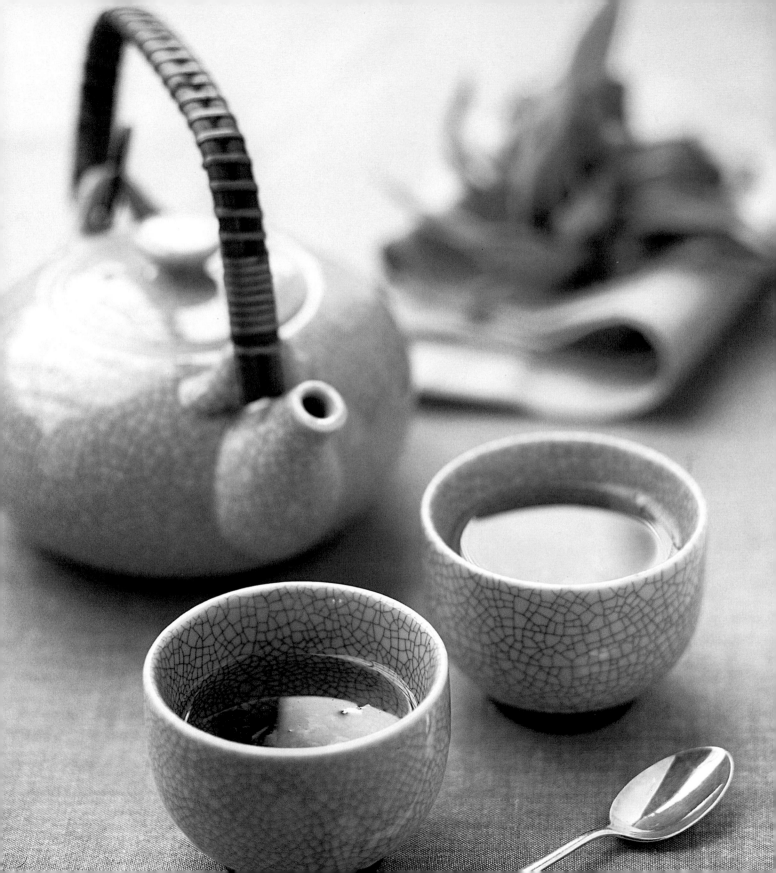

Thyme, Elecampane, and Cardamom Tea

This tea is great for persistent wet coughs, as it encourages the removal of mucus built up in the lungs. Thyme makes an excellent expectorant and antispasmodic, at the same time relaxing bronchial constriction in the lungs. The fragrant volatile oil of thyme is a good antiseptic and anti-microbial. Elecampane facilitates the removal of mucus from the lungs by stimulating and inducing coughing. Cardamom is warming to the body and adds flavor.

Makes 1 cup (8 fl oz/250 ml)
serves 1

1 teaspoon shredded dried elecampane root
1 cup (8 fl oz/250 ml) water
1 teaspoon dried thyme leaves and/or flowers
pinch of ground cardamom

Soak the elecampane in the water overnight. Strain and then heat the liquid in a small saucepan until almost boiling. Add the thyme, remove from heat, cover, and let steep for 5–10 minutes. Pour through a strainer into a cup, stir in the cardamom, and drink hot.

Drink up to 3 cups a day.

Note: If you find that drinking this tea stimulates too much coughing, replace elecampane with marshmallow root, which is soothing and relaxes irritating coughs.

Oat Straw and Alfalfa Tea

This tea is ideal if you have been sick for some time, have little appetite, and don't feel quite yourself. It can be taken any time you are feeling rundown. Oat straw has a bland taste, but it strengthens the nervous system and is rich in silica and calcium. Alfalfa is rich in iron, vitamin A, B, C, D, and E, and is particularly good for convalescence.

Makes 2 cups (16 fl oz/500 ml)
serves 2–3

3 tablespoons dried oat straw
1 tablespoon alfalfa seed
2 cups (16 fl oz/500 ml) water

Combine the oat straw, alfalfa seed, and water in a small saucepan. Bring to a boil over high heat. Reduce heat to medium-low, cover, and then simmer for 20 minutes, or until reduced by one-third. Strain, then drink.

Drink 1 cup of this tea every 3 hours for 2–4 weeks.

Note: You can add $1/2$ teaspoon of ground licorice root to give this tea extra benefits for the adrenal glands, and to improve its taste.

Caution: Licorice should be avoided if you have high blood pressure. Avoid oat straw if you are sensitive to gluten or have coeliac disease.

Right: Oat Straw and Alfalfa Tea

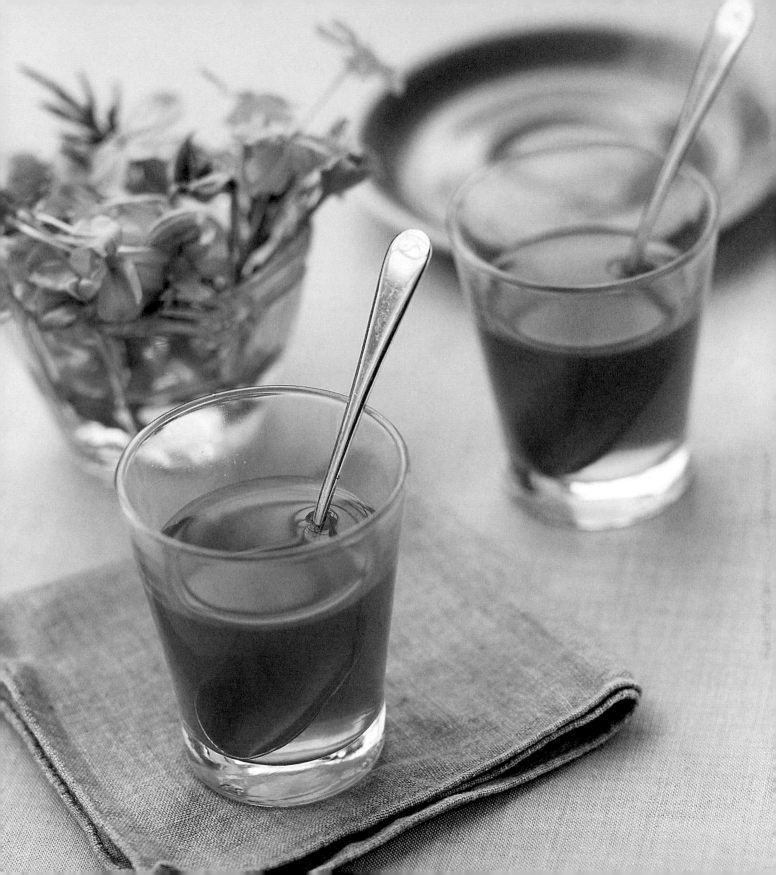

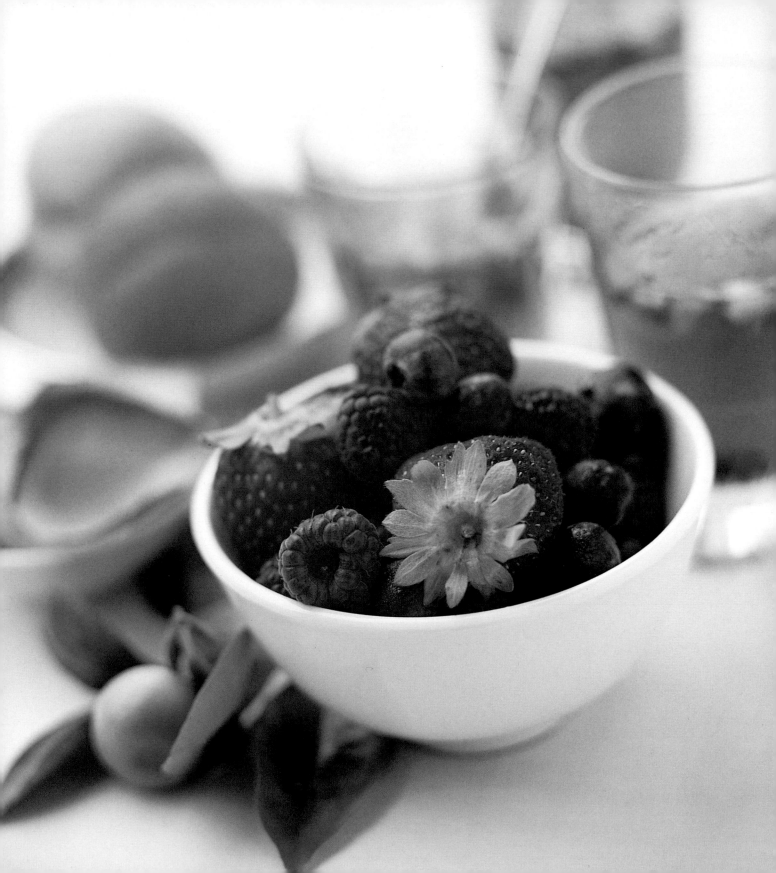

fRUIT TEA BLENDS

Tea shops shelves are filled with colorful canisters with wonderful surprises inside them. I was invited to take a look inside one of the canisters, and as it was opened I was engulfed by the magical aroma of dried strawberries. I don't think I'll ever forget that fragrance. And that's one of the delightful pleasures of making a fruit tea: the aroma is unforgettable.

Fruit teas are made from the fruits of various trees, plants, and shrubs. Fruits such as berries, rosehips (the ripe fruit of the rose), and citrus are the varieties most often used. They can be used medicinally, depending on the variety, or enjoyed just for their tangy flavor.

In Chinese medicine, the sweet taste of fruit is associated with weight gain and the stomach. Fruits are considered yin, with cold and damp. The orange, for example, native to China before it spread to Arabia and the rest of the Mediterranean, is used in Chinese medicine as a digestive stimulant and to improve qi (the flow of energy), as well as a treatment for phlegm, coughs, and insomnia.

Sacred hawthorn berries, with their slightly sweet flavor, were known as mother of the heart because they work on the cardiac actions within the body. They can relax the heart and arteries, decreasing blood pressure. Hawthorn berries were added to bread in England during World War I to bring down the blood pressure of the population.

Fruits are usually high in vitamin C and bioflavonoids, which make them great antioxidants. Berries, with their deep purple colors, are great for the eyes; they improve eyesight, relieve tired, red eyes, and constrict the blood vessels in the eye, making them look clear and vibrant. Drinking a good strong cup of berry tea once or twice daily will work wonders.

To make your own fruit tea, the fruit needs to be dried. Pick or select your fruit when it is just ripe. Slice the fruit, then spread it evenly out on a drying surface and remember to turn it over often to prevent mold from forming on it. (See page 103 for more details on drying fruit.)

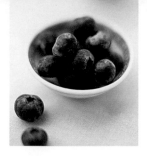

Bilberry and Green Tea

Bilberry and green tea are both very strong antioxidants. Bilberry has long been used therapeutically for glaucoma and other eye-related diseases. Bilberry is diuretic and astringent, and has a cooling and drying effect on the body. It also improves the production of insulin, which is useful in the treatment of adult onset diabetes. The flavor of green tea is masked by the flavor of the bilberry; however, its digestive-enhancing qualities are still present.

Makes 1 cup (8 fl oz/250 ml)
serves 1

1 teaspoon dried bilberries
¹/₂ teaspoon green tea leaves
1 cup (8 fl oz/250 ml) boiling water

Combine the bilberry and green tea leaves in a warmed small ceramic or glass teapot or cup. Add the boiling water, cover, and let steep for 5–10 minutes. Strain, then drink hot to warm.

Hawthorn Berry, Lemon Rind and Lime Blossom Tea

This tea has a slight sweet-to-sour taste that warms the body. Tests in Japan show that hawthorn berries have positive cardiac effects, reducing blood pressure and the heart rate. It is also useful in the treatment of edema and dyspnea (shortness of breath). Lemon rind contains citrus flavonoids that improve varicose veins and are antihistaminic. Lime blossoms also have cardiac properties, reducing blood pressure and helping nervous disorders.

Makes 2 cups (16 fl oz/500 ml)
serves 2–3

1 tablespoon dried hawthorn berries
¹/₂ teaspoon grated lemon zest (rind)
1 tablespoon dried lime blossom
2 cups (16 fl oz/500 ml) boiling water

Place the hawthorn berries, lemon zest and lime blossom in a warmed ceramic or glass teapot. Add the boiling water and let steep for 10–15 minutes. Strain, then drink hot or cool.

Drink one to two cups of the tea each day.

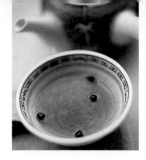

Orange, Cinnamon, and Peach Tea

Orange and orange zest have been used to flavor food and drinks for decades. Orange is used as a stomachic (calming and relaxing to the digestive system). The flavonoids in orange are also anti-inflammatory, antibacterial, and antifungal. Cinnamon is a gentle circulatory stimulant, as it increases blood flow, thus warming the hands and feet. It has been used for thousands of years to treat nausea and vomiting, and it is also a digestive healing herb. Peach adds a delightful color and flavor to this aromatic brew. If dried peaches are not available, substitute dried apricots.

Makes 2 cups (16 fl oz/500 ml)
serves 2–3

1 teaspoon grated fresh orange zest (rind)
1 teaspoon ground cinnamon
1 tablespoon chopped dried peach
2 cups (16 fl oz/500 ml) boiling water

Combine the orange zest, cinnamon, and peach in a warmed ceramic or glass teapot. Add the boiling water, cover, and let steep for 5 minutes.

Note: You can strain this tea to drink as a refresher during summer or as a digestive after a heavy meal.

Juniper and Cranberry Juice Tea

Juniper, with its pungent, bittersweet flavor, has long been used as an antiseptic that flushes and cleanses the entire urinary system. It is useful in treating cystitis, gout, and other types of rheumatism. Cranberry has a long history of soothing and healing urinary mucus. It makes acid urine less acidic, thus decreasing the burning pain associated with cystitis.

Makes 2 cups (16 fl oz/500 ml)
serves 2–3

2 teaspoons dried juniper berries
1 cup (8 fl oz/250 ml) boiling water
1 cup (8 fl oz/250 ml) cranberry juice

Put the juniper berries in a warmed ceramic or glass teapot. Add the boiling water, cover, and let steep for 10 minutes. Allow to cool and then combine with the cranberry juice.

Drink 1 cup twice daily.

Caution: Women who are pregnant should avoid juniper, as it is a uterine stimulant. Anyone suffering kidney disease should also avoid juniper.

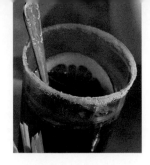

Lemon, Aniseed, and Fennel Seed Tea

Lemon juice and its zest are natural antimicrobials. Aniseed drinks were once a popular remedy for colds and flu. Both aniseed and fennel are lung-cleansing tonics, and they are given to women after delivery to encourage milk flow and to reduce colic in babies. Both have a slight licorice flavor. Fennel seeds have a reputation for suppressing the appetite if chewed before meals, and they also make an excellent breath freshener.

Makes 2 cups (16 fl oz/500 ml)
serves 2–3

1–2 teaspoons grated lemon zest (rind)
1 teaspoon aniseed
1–2 teaspoons fennel seeds
2 cups (16 fl oz/500 ml) boiling water

Combine the lemon zest, aniseed, and fennel seeds in a warmed ceramic or glass teapot. Add the boiling water, cover, and let steep for 10 minutes. Strain, then drink hot.

Drink 2–3 cups of this tea each day.

Lemon and Mint Tea

Lemon and mint tea is appropriate during the winter months as a warming tonic on a cold day. The lemon soothes sore throats and helps relieve colds. The rich vitamin C content in lemon helps combat colds and flu, while warming the body when drunk hot. Lemon and mint are both digestives, and can be taken after a heavy meal to aid digestion.

Makes 1 cup (8fl oz/250ml)
serves 1

1 teaspoon dried peppermint leaf
1 cup (8 fl oz/250 ml) boiling water
2 teaspoons lemon juice
honey to taste

Put the dried peppermint leaves in a warmed small ceramic or glass teapot or cup. Add the boiling water, cover, and let steep for 5 minutes. Strain, then add the lemon juice and honey.

Drink 2–3 cups a day for a week if you have a cold or a sore throat. Drink 1 cup after a heavy meal to relieve indigestion.

Black Currant and Cardamom Tea

Black currant is widely used to flavor food and as an ingredient in cereals and mixed dried nuts. High in vitamin C, the purplish-black fruits are used to treat diarrhea due to their high tannin content. Cardamom, native to India and Sri Lanka, is widely used as a culinary spice in foods such as curries, and it is commonly used to flavor Turkish coffee. It has antispasmodic activity, is calming to the digestive system, and is stimulating to the body.

Makes 1 cup (8 fl oz/250 ml)
serves 2–3

1 teaspoon dried black currants
¼ teaspoon ground cardamom
1 cup (8 fl oz/250 ml) boiling water

Combine the black currants and cardamom in a warmed ceramic or glass teapot. Add the boiling water, cover, and let steep for 5 minutes. Strain, then drink hot.

  Drink 1–2 cups a day, as required.

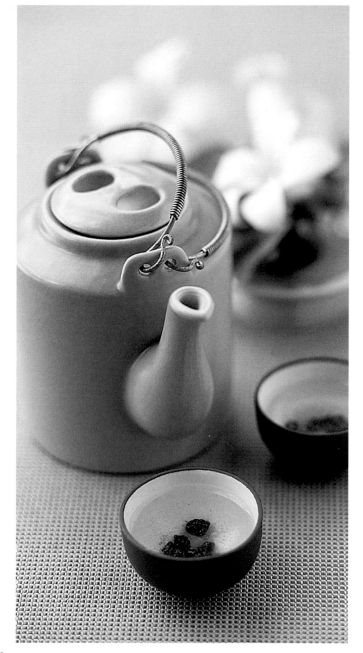

Right: Black Currant and Cardamom Tea

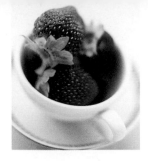

Dried Strawberry and Apple Tea

This tea can be drunk simply for pleasure as the taste and aroma are lovely. Strawberry is also mildly astringent, and is a diuretic. Both strawberries and apples are high in vitamin C.

Makes 1 cup (8 fl oz/250 ml)
serves 1

1 teaspoon chopped dried strawberry
1 teaspoon chopped dried apple
1 cup (8 fl oz/250 ml) boiling water

Combine the strawberry and apple in a warmed small ceramic or glass teapot or cup. Add the boiling water, cover, and let steep for 10 minutes. Drink hot, straining it first, if you like.

Hibiscus and Elderberry Tea

These two fruits are packed with vitamin C and anti-microbial properties. It is used medicinally to treat coughs, fever, and painful menstruation. Elderberry has long been used in England in making pies, preserves, and syrups. It is a decongestant and a tonic to the mucous membranes.

Makes 2 cups (16 fl oz/500 ml)
serves 2–3

1 tablespoon dried hibiscus calyces
1 tablespoon fresh or 2 teaspoons dried elderberries
2 cups (16 fl oz/500 ml) boiling water

Combine the hibiscus and elderberries in a warmed ceramic or glass teapot. Add the boiling water, cover, and let steep for 10 minutes. Strain, then drink hot.

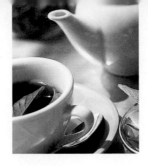

Raspberry and Hibiscus Tea

The leaves of the raspberry plant have long been used to treat women, especially during pregnancy. It is used to relieve morning sickness and prepare the uterus for birth, as well as for tonifying and strengthening the cervix. Its astringent taste is due to tannins. The tannin content in raspberry relieves diarrhea, and makes raspberry tea a good gargle for mouth and throat infections. Hibiscus, with its citrus taste and bright red color, makes this a beautiful and flavorful tea.

Makes 1 cup (8 fl oz/250 ml)
serves 1

1 teaspoon dried raspberry leaves and/or berries
1/2 teaspoon dried hibiscus calyces
1 cup (8 fl oz/250 ml) boiling water

Combine the raspberry and hibiscus in a warmed small ceramic or glass teapot or cup. Add the boiling water, cover, and let steep for 10 minutes. Strain, then drink hot.

Drink up to 2 cups a day for the last 3 months before the birth of a baby to prepare for an easy delivery, and drink during labor to assist the birth.

Vitex and Bilberry Tea

The plant *Vitex agnus-castus* has a pretty whirl of purple flowers and produces a lifesaving fruit that many women swear by for relieving premenstrual tension. Vitex will also increase lactation for nursing mothers. It is best taken first thing in the morning, as it works by regulating the pituitary gland. (If you suffer from PMS, you should also remove all caffeine-containing foods from your diet, as caffeine increases tension, worry, and anxiety.) Bilberry strengthens small blood vessels and is rich in bioflavonoids (antioxidants). This deep-purple tea is pretty when brewed in a glass teapot.

Makes 2 cups (16 fl oz/500 ml)
serves 2–3

1 tablespoon chopped dried vitex berries
2 teaspoons chopped dried bilberries
2 cups (16 fl oz/500 ml) boiling water

Combine the vitex and bilberries in a warmed small ceramic or glass teapot. Add the boiling water, cover, and let steep for 5–10 minutes. Strain, then drink hot.

Drink up to 2 cups a day.

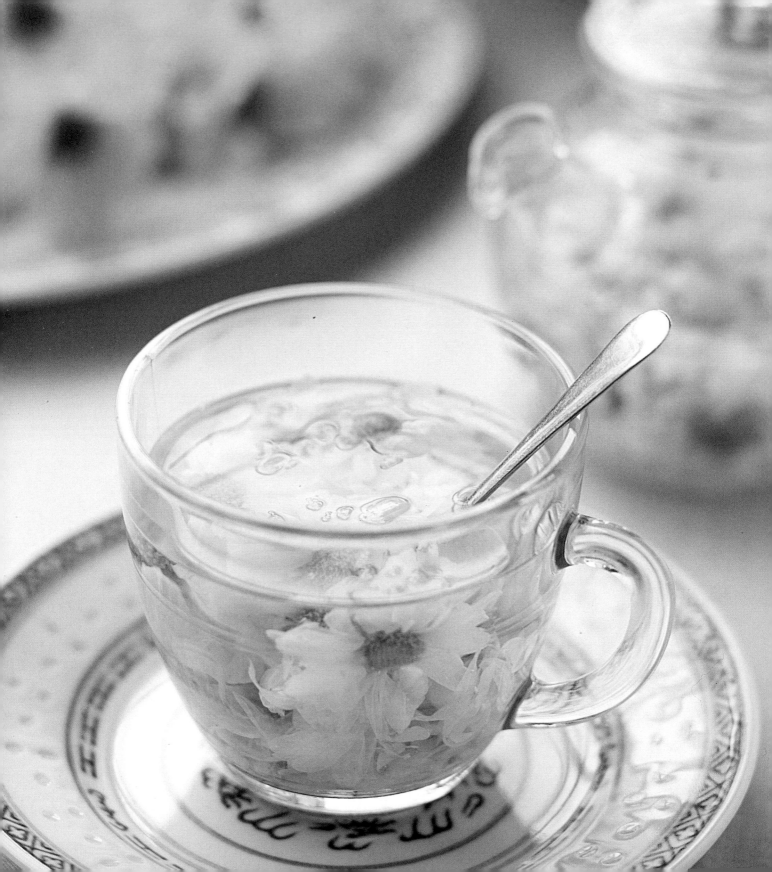

Exotic Floral Blends

floral teas are ideal to brew in a glass teapot. The colour of the petals will surprise your guests and so will the flavors of the flowers.

Flowers add serenity and peace to homes and workplaces, and can bring a smile to the face in seconds. Both because of their beauty and their fragility, they have been given as tokens of love and as offerings of worship to the gods throughout human history.

Flowers are highly regarded medicinally, and are used extensively to treat a variety of ailments, both in Chinese and Western herbalism. When dried correctly, flowers should retain their original color—discard if they do not. Chinese herbalists granulate some of their floral teas in a freeze-drying process. Sweetened chrysanthemum granules, for example, can be bought freeze-dried in little sachets, and they make a very refreshing tea that helps to soothe and nourish the eyes.

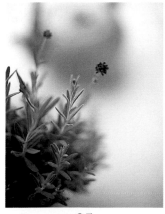

Left: Chrysanthemum and Ginger Tea

95

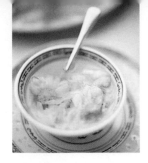

Chrysanthemum and Ginger Tea

Chrysanthemum is both sweet and bitter, and has a slightly cooling effect on the body. As a result, it is wonderful to drink on its own on hot, stuffy days. Mixed with ginger, however, the effect is counterbalanced, as ginger warms the body. Chrysanthemum tea can be well tolerated during fevers and headaches, it improves eyesight and can lower blood pressure. The yellow daisy-like flowers are used extensively in China as a poultice for sore, red eyes. Ginger adds a spicy flavor and assists fever treatment. It also flushes toxins caused by arthritis, and decreases pain and inflammation.

Makes 2 cups (16 fl oz/500 ml)
serves 2–3

1 tablespoon dried chrysanthemum flowers
1–2 teaspoons peeled and grated fresh ginger
2 cups (16 fl oz/500 ml) boiling water

Combine the chrysanthemum and ginger in a warmed ceramic or glass teapot. Add the boiling water, cover, and let steep for 10 minutes. Strain into a cup and drink hot.

Drink 1 cup of this tea every hour for fever, headaches, and arthritic pain.

Honeysuckle and Chamomile Tea

The honeysuckle is known for its delightful nectar. It is also considered a symbol of devotion. Honeysuckle is one of the most highly regarded Chinese herbs for promoting detoxification and cleansing of the body. It is used to treat fever and inflammation, to reduce blood pressure, and as an expectorant for coughs. It is also said to reduce freckles. Chamomile is a relaxing digestive that soothes and relaxes the whole body. This is just the tea to have after a stressful day.

Makes 1 cup (8 fl oz/250 ml)
serves 1

2 teaspoons dried honeysuckle flowers
1 teaspoon dried chamomile flowers
1 cup (8 fl oz/250 ml) boiling water

Combine the honeysuckle and chamomile in a warmed small ceramic or glass teapot. Add the boiling water, cover, and let steep for 10 minutes. Strain, then drink hot.

Note: To help reduce freckles, make a strong infusion of 1 cup (8 fl oz/250 ml) of crushed honeysuckle flowers (use fresh flowers if available) to 2 cups (16 fl oz/500 ml) of boiling water. Infuse for 15 minutes. Bathe face regularly in the infusion and/or add infusion to bath water.

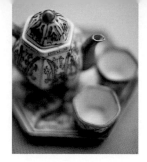

Elder Flower, Yarrow, and Clove Tea

The elder tree produces batch after batch of creamy white flowers that have a mucilaginous property when taken internally, coating and soothing the throat. The strong decongestant effect of these flowers makes elder valuable for treating colds and chills. But beware if planting; once an elder takes root, little elders will pop up everywhere. Yarrow is a small plant that bears white or purple umbrella-shaped flowers with a distinct odor and flavor. Yarrow is traditionally used as a steptic (to stop bleeding), due to its ability to strengthen blood vessels. Both these plants grow easily in backyards and are great for relieving flu symptoms. Cloves add flavor and increase the warming actions of the elder and yarrow.

Makes 2 cups (16 fl oz/500 ml)
serves 2–3

2–3 tablespoons chopped fresh elder flowers
1–2 tablespoons chopped fresh yarrow flowers
1/2 teaspoon ground cloves
2 cups (16 fl oz/500 ml) boiling water

Combine the elder flowers, yarrow flowers and cloves in a warmed ceramic or glass teapot. Add the boiling water, cover, and let steep for 10–15 minutes. Strain, then drink hot.

Drink 1 cup 3 times a day for colds and influenza.

Mallow and Peppermint Tea

Mallow was known as a cure-all in the 16th century. It has the ability to increase mothers' breast milk, to relieve sore, swollen breasts, and to soothe urinary tract infections. Mallow has a slightly astringent taste and can be applied externally to soothe weeping eczema, boils, and abscesses. Mallow flowers and leaves are used for coughs, sore throats, and emphysema. Peppermint, with its aromatic menthols, lends a stimulating flavor to this floral tea. It absorbs wind and is an excellent carminative; it also stops nausea and vomiting.

Makes 1 cup (8 fl oz/250 ml)
serves 1

1 teaspoon dried mallow flowers and/or leaves
1/2 teaspoon crumbled dried peppermint leaves
1 cup (8 fl oz/250 ml) boiling water

Combine the mallow and peppermint in a warmed small ceramic or glass teapot. Add the boiling water, cover, and let steep for 10 minutes. Strain, then drink hot.

Mullein and Angelica Tea

The yellow flowers of the mullein plant have been used to treat tuberculosis and other chest conditions, such as bronchitis, asthma, and whooping cough. An oil made from the flowers is used to treat hemorrhoids and ear infections. Mullein is best for treating dry, hard coughs. Angelica has been used for years as a sweet. It has warming medicinal properties and produces green-white flowers with a pleasant scent. The pretty flowers combine with mullein to make a relaxing expectorant and carminative. Honey may be added to taste, if desired.

Makes 1 cup (8 fl oz/250 ml)
serves 1

2 teaspoons mullein flowers, leaves and/or seeds
1 teaspoon angelica flowers, leaves, root, and/or seeds
1 cup (8 fl oz/250 ml) boiling water

Combine the mullein and angelica in a warmed small ceramic or glass teapot or cup. Add the boiling water, cover, and let steep for 20 minutes. Strain, then drink hot.

Drink up to 3 cups of this tea each day during an illness.

Lavender and Marshmallow Tea

Lavender has many therapeutic properties that help to relax the body during stressful situations. Aromatic lavender tea can help with problems such as headaches, low spirits, muscle tension, and nervous debility. Taking an infusion of lavender after a hard day at home or work can carry your worries away. It can also induce a peaceful, blissful slumber for those who have trouble falling asleep. As an infusion, it combines well with rosemary, skullcap, or chamomile. Lavender's purple-flowering blossoms have long been picked, dried, and placed in cupboards as sachets, or used to deter insects. Marshmallow has delicate pink flowers and is hard to find commercially, but it can be grown at home. It has a cool, moist, sweet character and is an effective, yet gentle cough expectorant.

Makes 2 cups (16 fl oz/250 ml)
serves 2–3

2 teaspoons lavender flowers and/or leaves
2 teaspoons marshmallow flowers, leaves and/or root
2 cups (16 fl oz/500 ml) boiling water

Combine the lavender and marshmallow in a warmed ceramic or glass teapot. Add the boiling water, cover, and let steep for 10 minutes. Strain, then drink hot.

Drink up to 3 cups a day if needed.

Right: Lavender and Marshmallow Tea

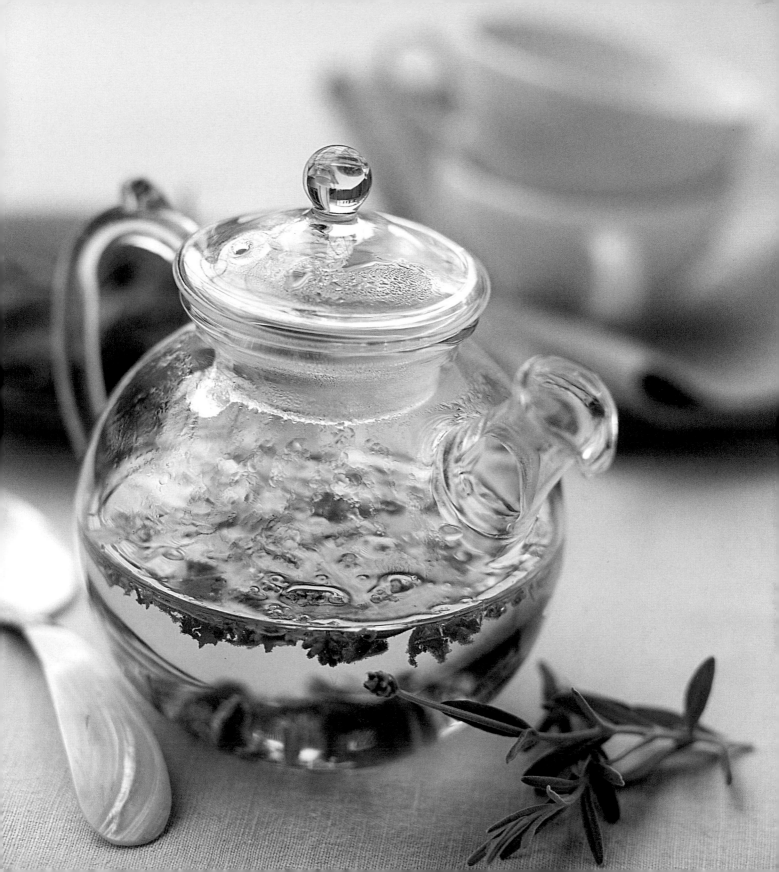

Rose Petal, Hibiscus, and Orange Zest Tea

The rose has a long history of medicinal use; its Latin name, *Rosa canina*, was given to it because of its history of being used to treat dog bites. An old herbal publication, *Askham's Herbal* (1550AD), says "Drye roses put to ye nose to smell do comforte the braine and the heart and quenche sprite." Chinese herbalists use rose petals as a blood tonic and to stimulate the liver. Hibiscus and the orange zest add a tangy flavor and vitamin C to this tea, making it a good winter beverage for colds and flus.

Makes 1 cup (8 fl oz/250 ml)
serves 1

2 teaspoons fresh rose petals
1 teaspoon dried hibiscus calyces
$^1/_2$ teaspoon grated orange zest (rind)
1 cup (8 fl oz/250 ml) boiling water

Combine the rose petals, hibiscus and orange zest in a warmed small ceramic or glass teapot or cup. Add the boiling water, cover, and let steep for 10 minutes. Strain, then drink hot.
  Drink 1 to 2 cups of the tea each day.

Yarrow and Cinnamon Tea

Yarrow is one of the best blood-vessel tonics there is. It improves venous return and fluid retention, and it is also valued as a treatment for colds and flu. Yarrow dilates blood vessels, thus decreasing blood pressure and improving blood flow throughout the body, especially for intermittent claudication. The flowers are antiallergic and expel heat from the body by causing sweating. Their bitter taste can be masked with the pleasant flavor of cinnamon, which also acts as an aromatic astringent, heating the body in cold temperatures. Cinnamon has been used for thousands of years to ease nausea and vomiting.

Makes 1 cup (8 fl oz/250 ml)
serves 1

2 teaspoons chopped fresh yarrow flowers
$^1/_4$ teaspoon ground cinnamon
1 cup (8 fl oz/250 ml) boiling water

Combine the yarrow and cinnamon in a warmed small ceramic or glass teapot or cup. Add the boiling water, cover, and let steep for 5–10 minutes. Strain, then drink hot.
  Drink up to 3 cups a day.

Right: Yarrow and Cinnamon Tea

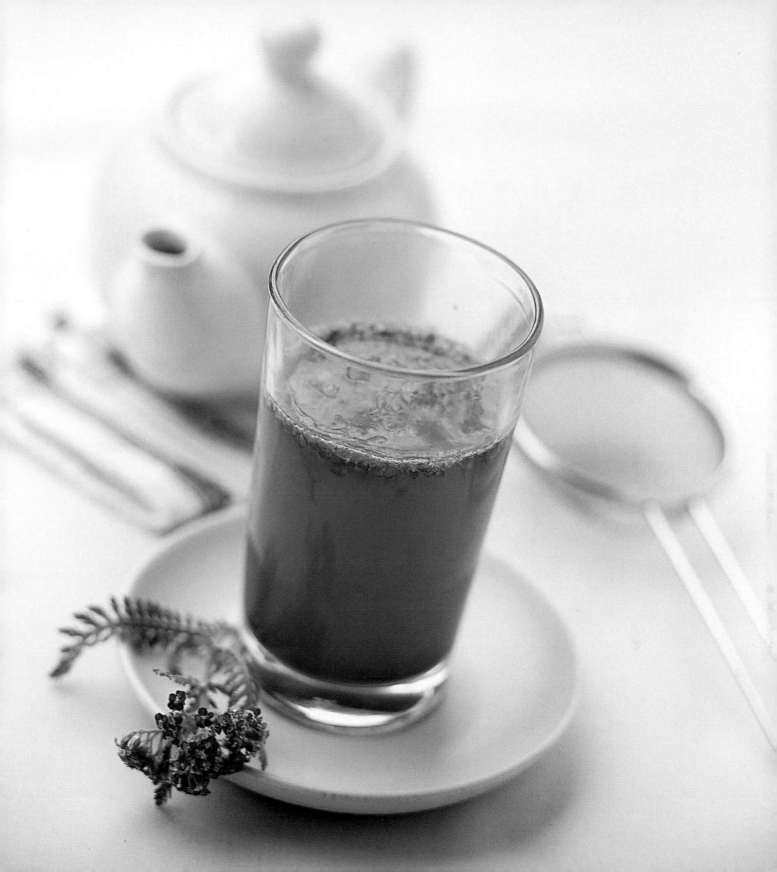

Tea from Your Garden

Many of the plants used to make tea are easy to grow. Most are hardy and grow well. When purchasing plants, make sure you buy the correct species by checking the Latin names. A good pictorial book will help to identify them. Some plants to grow at home include:

Trees

Elder (*Sambucus nigra*)

Ginkgo (*Ginkgo biloba*)

Hibiscus (*Hibiscus rosa-sinensis*)

Mulberry (*Morus nigra*)

Rose (*Rosa* spp.)

Tea (*Camellia sinensis*)

Small Plants, Shrubs and Bushes

Calendula (*Calendula officinalis*)

Chamomile (German) (*Matracaria recutita*)

Dandelion (*Taraxacum officinalis*)

Echinacea (*Echinacea* spp.)

Fennel (*Foeniculum vulgare*)

Feverfew (*Tanacetum parthenium*)

Globe artichoke (*Cynara scolymus*)

Ginger (*Zingiber officinale*)

Hawthorn (*Crataegus oxycanthoides*)

Juniper (*Juniper communis*)

Lavender (*Lavendula angustifolia*)

Lemon verbena (*Lippia citriodora*)

Nasturtium (*Tropaeolum majus*)

Passionflower (*Passiflora incarnata*)

Peppermint (*Mentha x piperita*)

Ribwort (*Plantago major*)

Rosemary (*Rosemarinus officinalis*)

Sage (*Salvia officinalis*)

Strawberry (*Fragaria vesca*)

St. John's Wort (*Hypericum perforatum*)

Sunflower (*Helianthus annus*)

Thyme (*thymus vulgaris*)

Valerian (*Valeriana officinalis*)

Yarrow (*Achillea millefolium*)

Harvesting

Harvest the uppermost parts of a plant on a dry day, just after the morning dew has dried and before the heat of the sun, usually between 9 and 10 am.

When picking leaves, choose the top leaves on the outside of the bush or plant. They should be fully mature and bright green. Cut stems with sharp scissors or clippers. Strip off strong leaves by running your hand down the stem firmly but gently. For softer leaves, pick one at a time to prevent damage. Flowers are best picked just before or immediately after they begin to bloom.

Roots should be harvested in autumn or winter when the plant has gone dormant for winter. Dig a wide circle around the plant. then gently remove some of the roots. Don't harvest more than half the root or that will kill the tree or shrub. The exception is dandelion, which tends to multiply voraciously and can be pulled out whole.

Drying

Plants should be dried immediately after picking. Spread the leaves, flowers, or roots on a gauze or mesh tray so there is plenty of air circulation. Be sure to spread them evenly, as drying them too close together will cause mold. Longer-stemmed plants can be cut and tied in bunches, covered with a paper bag, then hung upside down to dry in a dark, open cupboard or well-ventilated shed.

The ideal temperature for drying is 90°F (25–35°C). Cover mesh trays with paper at night to prevent insect infestation. Leaves and flowers can also be dried in an oven at 100°F (38°C).

After drying, plants should retain much of their original color and be dry enough to crackle. This indicates that they have been dried correctly, with minimal loss of essential oils and medicinal value.

Storing

Put the herbs in dark, dry, airtight glass containers, and store away from heat and light. Label every container with the plant name and date stored. Dried herbs will keep for 1–2 years. Store them whole and crumble just before making tea or when using in cooking.

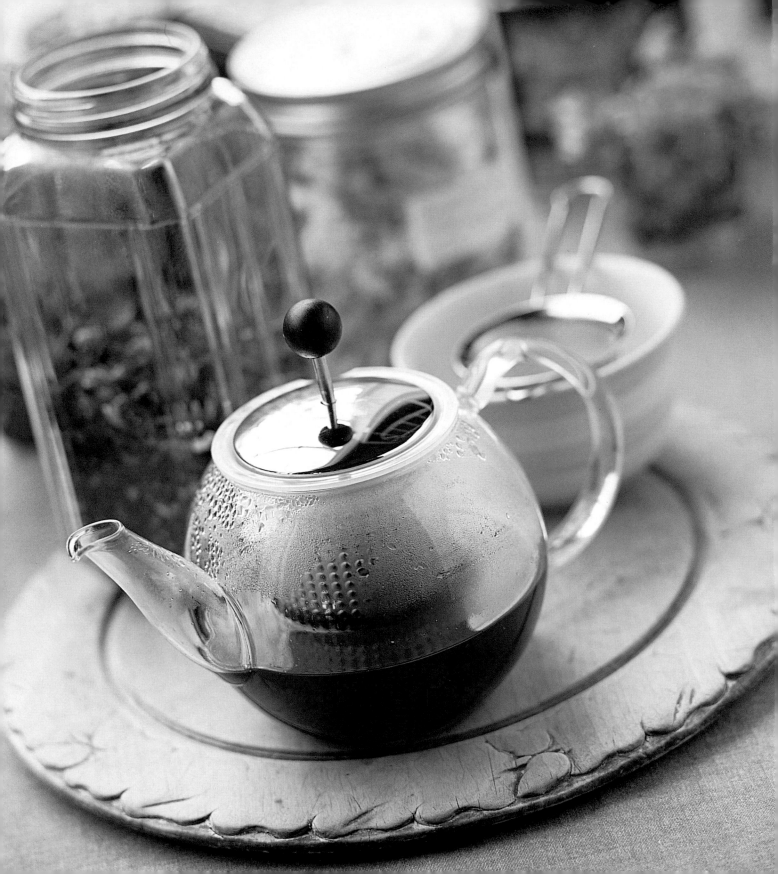

CREATING YOUR OWN SPECIAL BLENDS

Creating and experimenting with different tastes can be exciting. Some people like slightly bitter herbs. These can be teamed with nutmeg or cinnamon in an infused tea or simply brewed with lemongrass. Green teas tend to be slightly bitter, and the longer you brew the leaves in the hot water the more bitter they will become.

For sweet herbal teas, look for dried berries. These look attractive in glass teapots, as do flowers. The herb that is a must in the kitchen is licorice root. It blends well with all other herbs, yet it usually masks the flavor of other ingredients.

When brewing green teas, such as the fragrant Matcha, Sencha, or Gyokuro, never use a strainer. The leaf needs to be relaxed, or loose, so it can unfold, open up and release its flavor. The beauty behind this process is that each and every infusion will taste different. While some teas become lighter and milder with each brew, others become richer and fuller. If serving several people, pour a little tea into each cup, then come back and top them all up again. In China, tea is served from left to right, then from left to right again. This way everyone will get a similar-tasting tea. Return strained tea leaves to the teapot, and remember—do not leave any leaves soaking in hot water, strain it all off.

A very important point to remember is to never use a herb that you have not identified properly. Buy a good pictorial medicinal herb book that will help you identify various herbs or ask at your local plant nursery.

Keep all your herbs in jars, clearly labeled with the date, Latin and common names, along with what they are used for. Labeling will help remind you what works best for specific health problems. Once you have a selection of tea ingredients, you can display them in your kitchen so that you can offer choices to your guests. I have found over the years that guests are always keen to try one of my new brews. They tend to have their own special requests for a certain tea or herbal infusion. It definitely makes a pleasant change from the usual question, "Would you like tea or coffee?"

tea chart

Herb or Tea	Function	Health Benefit
Alfalfa (lucerne)	A relaxing nutritive, tonifying to the blood vessels	A tonic after blood loss and used to help reduce bleeding
Aniseed	An antiseptic and a cough expectorant; soothes abdominal cramps and spasms	Soothes coughs, chest infections, and colic with flatulence
Bilberry	Reduces blood sugar levels; an astringent and strong antioxidant for the eyes	Helps glaucoma, diabetes, and tired, bloodshot eyes
Black tea	A stimulant and a digestive; also an eye wash	Assists when you are feeling tired and out of sorts; gives you some get up and go
Buchu	A diuretic antiseptic to the urinary tract, with antibacterial activity	Use when there is blood and mucus in urine, indicating an infection in the urinary tract
Calendula	A strong anti-inflammatory, antiseptic, and antifungal; also a lymphatic cleanser	Helps whenever lymph glands are affected, as with glandular fever
Chamomile (German)	A bitter sedative, relaxing to the whole body; anti-inflammatory	Assists with insomnia and/or flatulence, cramping, and discomfort
Corn silk	Soothing to the urinary tract and respiratory system, diuretic and tonifying to the urinary tract	Helps with cystitis and bedwetting; prevents stone buildup in the kidneys
Dandelion	A diuretic rich in potassium, and also a digestive tonic, cleansing to rheumatic joints	Use for edema and indigestion, chronic skin conditions and arthritis
Elder	A diuretic, diaphoretic, and a gentle expectorant	For use when you have colds, flu, and sinus trouble, and for any catarrhal inflammation of the upper respiratory system
Eyebright	An anticatarrhal and anti-inflammatory, with an astringent effect	Specifically used for mucous membrane conditions, sinusitis, congestion, and phlegmy throat
Fennel	An antiseptic, antispasmodic expectorant that has relaxing actions on the digestive system	Relieves wind and cramping, and has a relaxing action on coughing; the oils are antiseptic for chest colds

Herb or Tea	Function	Health Benefit
Ginger	Warming to the body; an antinausea carminative and anti-inflammatory; diaphoretic (promotes a sweat)	For arthritis and tummy upsets, motion sickness, and fever
Ginseng	Increases and improves mental and physical performance	For the elderly and debilitated, to counteract memory loss, and to fortify after illness
Green tea	A digestive and a mild stimulant; nourishing and protective against cancer	Drink with meals to aid digestion; also acts as an antioxidant
Hawthorn	Decreases blood pressure and tonifies heart tissue; dilates peripheral blood vessels	Helps with hypertension, palpitations, and intermittent claudication
Hibiscus	An astringent with a citrus flavor; added to different tea blends	A tangy addition to other teas; a tonic for colds due to vitamin C content
Licorice	Known by herbalists as a panacea or cure-all, an anticatarrhal, an antiallergic anti–inflammatory, and an expectorant that soothes and heals digestive ulcers	Relieves coughs, colds, sore throats and flu. Assists in fever management, aids decongestion and soothes ulcers of the digestive tract
Oat Straw	Relaxing and nourishing to the nervous system, rich in calcium and fiber, helps alleviate rheumatic or back pain	Benefits a neurotic nervous personality, and alleviates debility and fatigue due to chronic nervousness; used in the bath for aches and pain
Rosemary	A warming digestive remedy and a relaxing antiseptic that promotes sweating; an antidepressant and brain stimulant	Aids indigestion, memory loss, low spirits, hair loss, and arthritis and related congestion
St John's wort	A sedative and tonic for the nervous system	For hysteria, low spirits, apathy, and fatigue from ill feelings
Thyme	A strong cleansing chest antiseptic; antimicrobial and carminative	Relieves bronchitis, asthma, gum and mouth infections, and bed-wetting
Yarrow	A peripheral vasodilator, tonic to all the blood vessels; an antispasmodic	Balances menstrual problems and manages fever and heavy bleeding; use topically as a poultice to heal wounds

glossary

Adaptogen: A herb that can help the body respond more favorably to stress by nurturing and strengthening that particular part of the body.

Adrenal glands: Glands situated at the top of each kidney that secrete the hormones adrenaline and nor adrenaline: the hormones responsible for the "fight or flight" response to sudden stress.

Antihistamine: A substance that stops histamine reaction by binding to histamine receptor sites in body tissue.

Anti-inflammatory: A substance that decreases or stops inflammation.

Antioxidant: A substance that inhibits destructive oxidation in the body; some examples are vitamins C and E, selenium and green tea.

Astringent: A substance that has a drying effect, tightening and toning the cells and mucous membranes.

Bioflavonoids: Plant pigments (usually yellow in color) also known as vitamin P. They include rutin, quercetin, and hesperidin, and they have potent anti-inflammatory actions and improve the absorption of vitamin C.

Bud: The unopened leaf at the very top of a tree/bush, sought after for its tenderness and sweetness.

Carminative: An herb that decreases flatulence and relaxes the muscles in the body by decreasing tension.

Cha: Japanese for "tea".

Chanoyu: Japanese for "hot water for tea".

Cystitis: An infection or inflammation of the urinary bladder.

Decongestant: An herb or remedy that removes mucus congestion from the body.

Dehydration: When the body is lacking in water.

Diuretic: A herb or remedy that increases urinary output.

Dyspnea: Shortness of breath and difficulty in breathing.

Dust: Powdery pieces of tea, less than 0.04 inch (1 mm) in length.

Edema: Fluid retention that results in swelling, usually of the limbs.

Emphysema: A disease of the alveoli in the lungs, where the alveoli are permanently expanded and inflamed by an overproduction of mucus, which causes difficulty in breathing.

Expectorant: An herb or remedy that increases the removal of mucus from the lungs.

Fermentation: When the tea leaves become oxidized, the cell structure is changed, and the leaf becomes darker, drier and richer in flavor.

Formosa: (Former name of Taiwan) an island off the coast of China that grows Oolong, Pouchong and black teas.

Glaucoma: A disease of the eye where there is increased pressure in the eye fluids, which results in a progressive loss of eyesight.

Gout: A painful inflammation, usually of the big toe or other joints, caused by uric acid buildup in the joints.

Insomnia: The inability to sleep.

Intermittent claudication: An initial symptom of arteriosclerosis, which manifests as pain, cramps or a tired feeling in the limbs, especially in the calf muscle.

Jaundice: An increase of bile in the blood, resulting in a yellowing of the skin and sclera (white sections) of the eyes, loss of appetite, and lethargy.

Magnesium: An important mineral in the body, responsible for muscle relaxation and contraction. It works closely with calcium.

Menopause: When a woman ceases to menstruate.

Mucilaginous: Refers to the nature of mucilage, i.e., various gummy secretions present in plants.

Mucus: A viscid fluid secreted by the inner lining of the digestive tract, glands, and lungs. During a disease state, it may be oversecreted and be present as phlegm in the respiratory system.

Mucous membranes: Membranes that line the whole digestive tract from mouth to anus, and other organs. They secrete mucus to coat and protect.

Palpitation: An abnormal throbbing of the heart that can be felt by the person.

Pan-fired: Green tea that has been steamed then rolled in woks or pans over charcoal. This process ensures even drying of the leaves, enhancing their quality and flavor.

Phytoestrogens: Plant compounds that have an estrogenic effect within the body.

Polyphenols: Chemical compounds found in certain substances, that have disinfective and antiseptic qualities.

Rolling: An action that releases essential oils in tea leaves.

Reflux: The back flow of food up the esophagus, usually caused by indigestion.

Steptic: A remedy that can stop bleeding.

Stomachic: A remedy that is nourishing and soothing to the digestive system.

Tannin: An astringent chemical found in some herbs and in the tea plant.

Tatami: A Japanese straw mat; laid on the floor during the tea ceremony.

Tip: The bud leaf on a tea plant.

Tonifying: The healing and improving of the function of organs or tissues.

Withering: The first stage in making black tea. It reduces moisture so that the leaf can be macerated (softened) or rolled.

Botanical Names

alfalfa (*Medicago sativa*)
angelica (*Angelica archangelica*)
aniseed (*Pimpinella anisum*)
astragalus (*Astragalus membranaceus*)
bilberry (*Vaccinium myrtilis*)
black cohosh (*Cimicifuga racemosa*)
black currant (*Ribes nigrum*)
buchu (*Barosima betulina*)
calendula (*Calendula officinalis*)
cardamom (*Elattaria cardamomum*)
chamomile (*Matracaria recutita*)
chickweed (*Stellaria media*)
chrysanthemum (*Chrysanthemum* x *morifolium*)
cinnamon (*Cinnamomum verum*)
clivers (*Galium aparine*)
clove (*Syzygium aromaticum*)
corn silk (*Zea mays*)
dandelion (*Taraxacum radix*)
echinacea (*Echinacea purpurea/angustifolia*)
elder (*Sambucus nigra*)
elderberry (*Sambucus nigra*)
elecampane (*Inula helenium*)
eyebright (*Euphrasia officinalis*)

fennel (*Foeniculum vulgare*)
ginger (*Zingiber officinale*)
golden rod (*Solidago virgaurea*)
gotu kola (*Centella asciatica*)
hawthorn (*Crataegus* spp.)
hibiscus (*Hibiscus rosa-sinensis*)
honeysuckle (*Lonicera japonica*)
hop (*Humulus lupulus*)
horehound (*Marribum vulgare*)
juniper (*Juniperus communis*)
Korean ginseng (*Panax ginseng*)
lavender (*Lavendula angustifolia*)
lemon (*Citrus limon*)
lemon balm (*Melissa officinalis*)
lemon grass (*Cymbogon citratus*)
licorice (*Glyccyrrhiza glabra*)
lime (*Tilia europea*)
mallow (*Malva sylvestris*)
marshmallow (*Althaea officinalis*)
meadow sweet (*Filipendula ulmaria*)
mullein (*Verbascum thapsus*)
nettle (*Urtica diocia*)
oak bark (*Quercus robur*)
oat straw (*Avena sativa*)

orange (*Citrus sinensis*)
passionflower (*Passiflora incarnata*)
peach (*Prunus persica*)
peppermint (*Mentha* x *piperita*)
plantain, see ribwort
raspberry (*Rubus idaeus*)
red clover (*Trifolium pratense*)
ribwort (*Plantago major*)
rose (*Rosa* spp.)
rosemary (*Rosmarinus officinalis*)
sage (*Salvia officinalis*)
Seville orange (*Citrus aurantium/Citrus reticulata*)
Siberian ginseng (*Eleutherococcus senticosus*)
skullcap (*Scutellaria lateriflora*)
St. John's wort (*Hypericum perforatum*)
strawberry (*Fragaria vesca*)
tea (*Camellia sinensis*)
thyme (*Thymus vulgarus*)
uva ursi (*Arctostophylos uva-ursi*)
valerian (*Valeriana officinalis*)
vervain (*Verbena officinalis*)
vitex (*Vitex agnus-castus*)
yarrow (*Achillea millefolium*)

ailments index

ingredients index

Recommended Reading

Burgess, Anthony, *The Book of Tea*, New York: Abbeville Press, 1992.

Gary and Zong Xiao-fan, *Chinese Medicinal Teas*, Boulder Colorado: Blue Poppy Press, 1996.

Lu, C. Henry, *Chinese Herbal Cures*, New York: Sterling Publishing, 1991.

Ody, Penelope, *The Complete Medicinal Herbal*, New York: DK Publishing 1993.

Perry, Sara, *The Book of Herbal Teas*, San Francisco: Chronicle Books, 1997.

Rosen, Diana, *Green Tea*, London: Souvenir Press, 2000.

Sach, Penelope, *On Tea and Healthy Living*, Sydney: Allen & Unwin, 1995.

Published in the United States by Periplus (HK) Ltd.
www.periplus.com

© Copyright 2001 Lansdowne Publishing Pty. Ltd.

Library of Congress Cataloguing-in-Publication Data is available.
ISBN 978-0-7946-5004-9

DISTRIBUTED BY
USA
Tuttle Publishing
364 Innovation Drive
North Clarendon, VT 05759-9436 U.S.A.
Tel: 1 (802) 773-8930, Fax: 1 (802) 773-6993
info@tuttlepublishing.com
www.tuttlepublishing.com

Japan
Tuttle Publishing
Yaekari Building, 3rd Floor
5-4-12 Osaki, Shinagawa-ku, Tokyo 141-0032
Tel: (81) 3 5437-0171, Fax: (81) 3 5437-0755
sales@tuttle.co.jp
www.tuttle.co.jp

Asia Pacific
Berkeley Books Pte. Ltd.
61 Tai Seng Avenue #02-12, Singapore 534167
Tel: (65) 6280-1330, Fax: (65) 6280-6290
inquiries@periplus.com.sg
www.periplus.com

Set in Giovanni on QuarkXPress
Printed in Singapore   1307CP

13 14 15 16   11 10 9 8

VEGETABLE CREATIONS

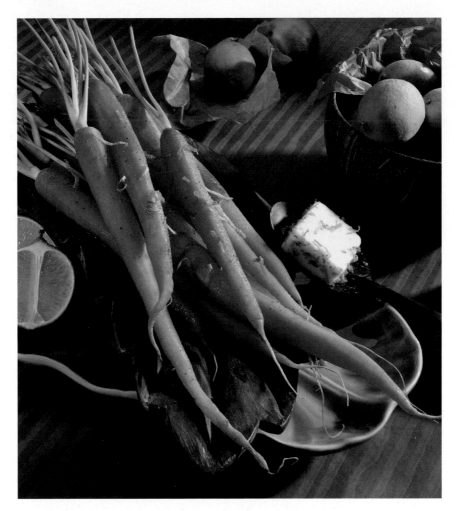

Cooking Arts Collection™

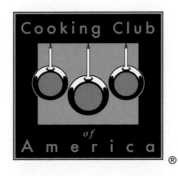

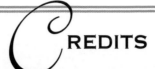

CREDITS

About the Author

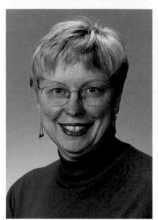

Mary Evans, founder of *Mary Evans Cooks*, has been involved in the culinary field for the past 20 years. A former cooking school director, she enjoys sharing her passion for food with others through cooking classes, developing recipes, and writing on a wide variety of food topics. Addicted to travel, she leads food-related tours in the U.S. and France. Her culinary background involves studies at La Varenne and Lenôtre. Mary is a member of the International Association of Culinary Professionals and Les Dames d'Escoffier.

VEGETABLE CREATIONS

Copyright ©2000 Cooking Club of America

Mike Vail, Vice President, Product and Business Development

Tom Carpenter, Director of Book Development

Dan Kennedy, Book Production Manager

Jen Guinea, Book Development Coordinator

Tad Ware & Company: Book Design and Production
Photography
Food Styling
Recipe Testing

2 3 4 5 6 7 8 / 02 01 00
ISBN 1-58159-105-5

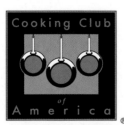

Cooking Club of America
12301 Whitewater Drive
Minnetonka, MN 55343

$\mathcal{T}$ABLE OF CONTENTS

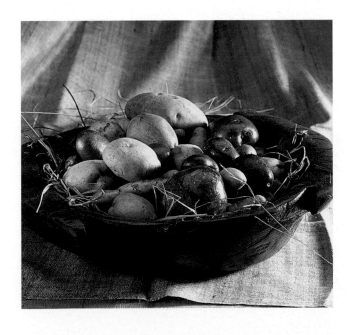

*I*NTRODUCTION

Let's play word association. Describe vegetables. What's the first word that comes to mind — colorful, flavorful, delicious, crunchy, healthy?

Carry those words with you the next time you visit the produce section of your supermarket or, better yet, your local farmers' market. Notice the vivid palette of colors glowing back at you. Feel the endless variety of textures these vegetables represent, from smooth to velvety, from firm to ripely yielding. Your enjoyment has begun and you haven't even made a purchase! Pick up a few favorites, but then add an unusual item or two to broaden your culinary horizons. If you've never cooked a parsnip before, now may be the time to try. Just turn to the side dish chapter for guidance. For added reinforcement, turn to the glossary section of this book and learn all the healthy benefits to some mighty tasty eating.

Now let's try a different exercise. Don't think about vegetables as something to fill up the holes on your plate. Instead, move them center stage and think of everything else as complementary. Many of the following recipes make vegetables the star of any course; you'll find an excellent assortment of appetizers, soups, main dishes and desserts, along with the more typical salads and side dishes. According to most health studies, eating vegetables contributes significantly to longevity. The food pyramid suggests three to five vegetable servings per day. Make produce the focus of your diet and you'll be amazed how great you feel.

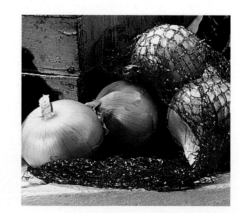

Along with fabulous recipes, this book includes a section on cooking techniques for recipe success, with some broader suggestions for adding life to any vegetable side dish. Check out some of the tools and gadgets that make cooking easier. The glossary sums up all the useful, factual information you need to know about vegetables; it also offers tips on how to select the best and freshest produce, and how to keep your vegetables at optimum quality once you've gotten them home.

Once you're hooked, try growing your own vegetables and herbs. Even the most limited space can accommodate a few pots in a sunny location. Try one tomato plant on the deck, terrace or patio, or a few herbs along a windowsill.

Introduce children to where food comes from by giving them the pleasure of watching things grow. They'll eat foods you never thought possible because they grew them. As an aside, "Eat your vegetables" is a sentence that should be banned from the English language. Said in a firm parental tone guaranteed to discourage even the most avid eater, it leaves many children marred well into adulthood with an unfortunate aversion to nature's best. Let them learn by example, and by helping in the selection and cooking process whenever possible.

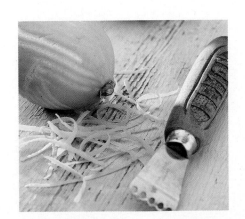

And remember that whatever stage of life you're at, vegetables are to be celebrated and savored. That's what *Vegetable Creations* is all about.

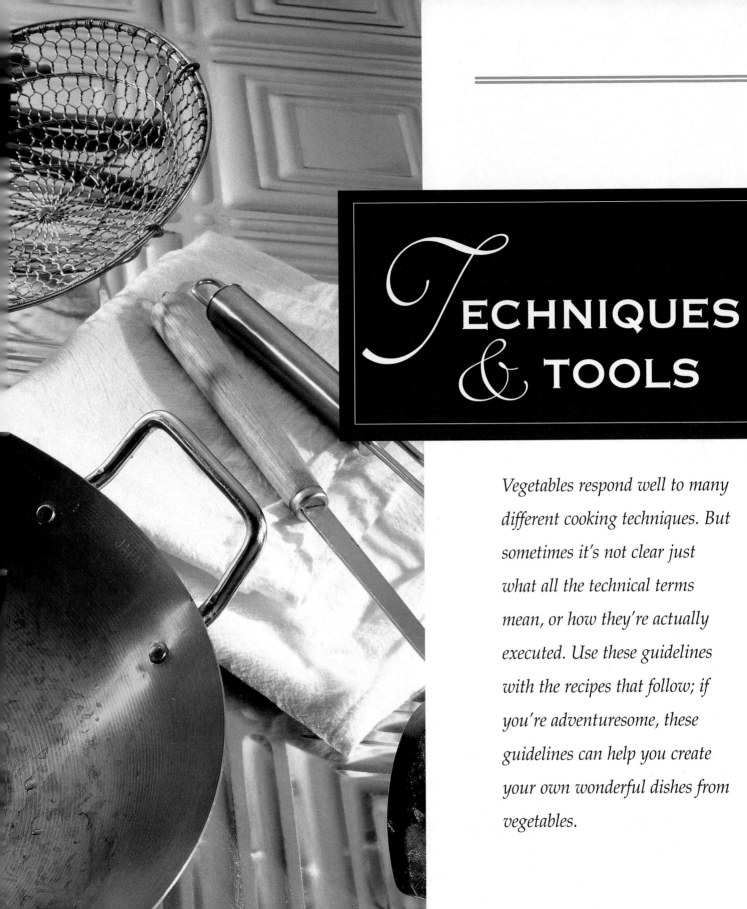

TECHNIQUES & TOOLS

Vegetables respond well to many different cooking techniques. But sometimes it's not clear just what all the technical terms mean, or how they're actually executed. Use these guidelines with the recipes that follow; if you're adventuresome, these guidelines can help you create your own wonderful dishes from vegetables.

BLANCH/PARBOIL

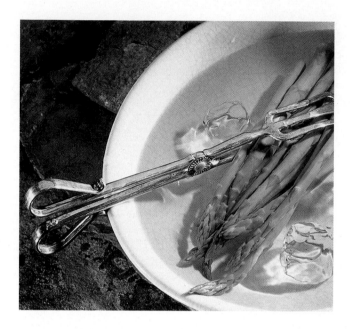

Blanching or parboiling involves dropping vegetables into a large quantity of rapidly boiling water for a short period of time. It is meant to partially, but not completely, cook the food being blanched.

There are several reasons to blanch. Sometimes cooks use this technique to set the color of a vegetable or make it more vivid. For example, the pea pods in *Spicy Pea Pod and Orange Salad* (page 55) take on fabulous color after their brief plunge in boiling water. Sometimes vegetables are blanched to make them more tender, as are the sugar snaps and asparagus in *Spring Sugar Snaps, Asparagus Spears and Radishes with Mint-Chive Dip* (page 39).

Try blanching or parboiling sometime when adding a vegetable such as broccoli to a salad, to make it more colorful and tender. Blanching is also necessary before freezing vegetables to retard enzyme action.

After blanching, drain vegetables and then, if small quantities are involved, run under cold water to avoid overcooking. For larger quantities, have a bowl of water with ice handy and plunge the drained, blanched vegetables into it.

BRAISE/STEW

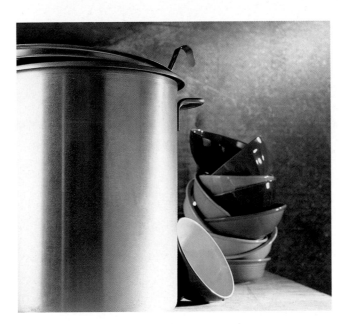

Braising is a term that describes the process of cooking a particular food slowly in a small amount of liquid. Stewing usually involves more than one food item, and often calls for more liquid.

These similar techniques use a covered or partially covered pot on top of the stove, in the oven or in a slow cooker. Cook food in this manner to either tenderize, add moisture or mingle flavors. Some examples are the *Braised Beans in Hoisin Sauce* (page 80), *Cauliflower and Garbanzo Bean Tagine* (page 105), *Indian Root Vegetable Curry* (page 109) and *Vegetarian Gumbo* (page 117), among others.

Also use these techniques when cooking tougher, leaner cuts of meats (with or without vegetables), or any time you want flavors to blend.

GRILL/BROIL

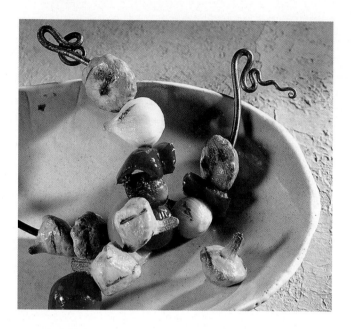

These techniques involve cooking food above or below a direct heat source. Both grilling and broiling produce similar results — quickly cooked food that is well-browned.

Because this is a dry cooking process, vegetables need to be brushed or sprayed with a bit of oil to keep them from losing their moisture while cooking. Grilled or broiled vegetables develop a slightly smoky or charred taste that complements certain dishes. Because the heat source is so intense, watch food carefully to avoid burning. Food should not be too thick or large when prepared in this manner or else it will not cook properly.

The recipe for *Black Bean, Corn and Green Chile Quesadillas* (page 25) cooks both the corn and the chiles in this way. Also try grilling or broiling for vegetables to serve with pasta or on top of pizza: Cut the vegetables into slices, cook until well-browned and cut into bite-size pieces.

$\mathcal{M}$ ICROWAVE

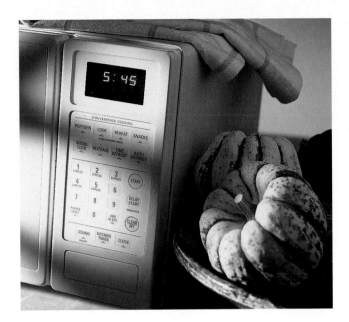

In general, vegetables cook very well in the microwave. Microwaves cook by moving the water molecules around in food, creating friction and thus generating heat. Most vegetables have a high moisture content and thus cook quickly and well. The resulting texture will be similar to steamed foods.

Because this technique requires little or no additional liquid, water-soluble vitamins are not washed away during the cooking process. While microwaving is not specified in any of the recipes in this book, try it when cooked vegetables are listed as ingredients. Corn, winter squash and sweet potatoes would be prime examples.

Because microwaves vary widely in wattages, refer to your owner's manual for proper cooking times. Do not microwave vegetables when browning is desired.

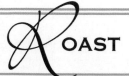OAST

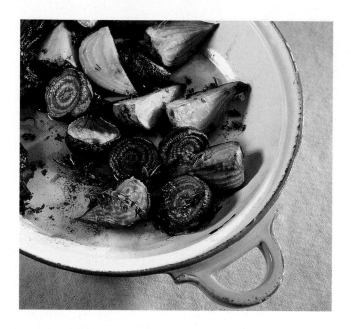

Roasting is a dry heat process that involves cooking food in the oven, using fairly high heat to promote browning. Although it is most often used for meats, roasting also caramelizes vegetables and gives them a richer taste. Roasting is used in the recipe for *Rich Vegetable Stock* (page 61).

Here's another idea. Try cutting up vegetables (most any will do), toss them with a bit of oil and place them in a fairly hot oven (400°F or so) for 30 to 45 minutes, stirring occasionally. Cut the larger vegetables into chunks before roasting. Serve these flavorful vegetables as a no-fuss side dish with lots of taste.

SAUTE/STIR-FRY

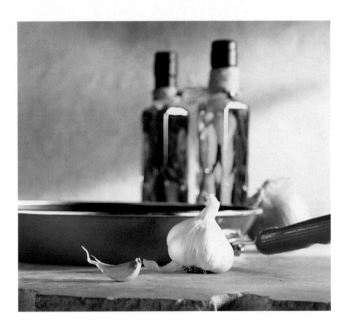

Both sautéing and stir-frying cook food quickly over a direct heat source, using a large cooking surface and a small amount of oil or fat.

Sautéing involves a skillet and is usually done over medium to medium-high heat. It takes a bit longer than stir-frying. Onion and garlic are often sautéed at the beginning of a recipe to quickly soften them and release their flavor.

Stir-fry in a wok over high heat; position the wok as close to the heat source as possible. Because the outer surface of food is cooked so quickly, it needs to be chopped, cut in strips or be relatively thin so that the interior will cook before the exterior burns. *Sesame Asparagus* (page 90) is a good example of wok cooking.

Use the stir-fry method for an easy, quick dinner. Here's how: Cut whatever vegetables you have on hand into strips. Do the same with a small amount of meat, if desired. Stir-fry the vegetables with a bit of oil, ginger and garlic; start by adding the vegetables that are a bit sturdier and need more cooking. Add a little water, if necessary, to finish the process by steaming. If adding meat, remove the vegetables, add a little more oil and quickly stir-fry the meat. Return the vegetables to the pan, adding a bit of bottled stir-fry sauce or oyster or hoisin sauce for flavor. Serve with rice.

SIMMER/BOIL

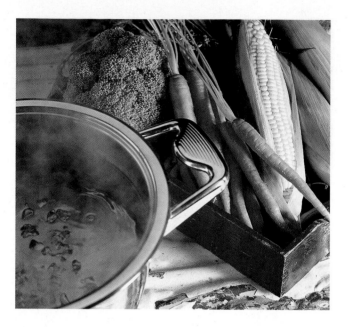

Simmering involves heating liquid until small bubbles form; boiling creates larger bubbles. Use low heat when simmering, medium heat or higher for boiling.

Because simmering is a gentler, slower cooking method, it is often used to avoid breaking apart food, and to concentrate taste. Soups are often simmered to release flavors into the cooking liquid. Broths and stocks do the same while evaporating some of the liquid to intensify the final product. Both stock recipes in this book rely on simmering, as do most of the soups.

Boiling cooks food more rapidly without releasing flavors. The green beans in *Green Beans Provencal* (page 83) are initially cooked this way. Sweet corn also cooks very well by boiling. Another advantage of boiling is that a large quantity of vegetables can be cooked very quickly.

$\mathcal{S}$TEAM

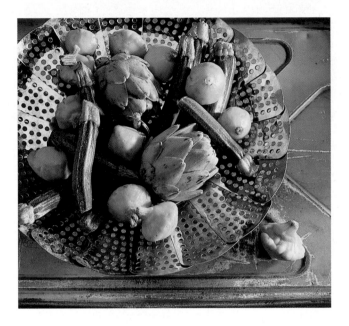

Steaming involves placing vegetables in a basket or insert with holes, then positioning the basket above a small amount of boiling water in a pan. The pan is covered and the resulting steam cooks the vegetables. Because the vegetables do not come in direct contact with the water, flavor and water-soluble vitamins are retained.

This technique is best for cooking relatively small amounts of vegetables simply and quickly. This is an easy way to cook vegetables simply for side dishes. Use this method to cook an accompaniment to an elaborate dish, for example, where anything but a plain vegetable would compete for attention.

USEFUL TOOLS

A good tool is an enormous asset for any kind of endeavor. Cooking is no exception. Here's a list of important tools and gadgets designed to make your vegetable creations even better, and your life in the kitchen easier.

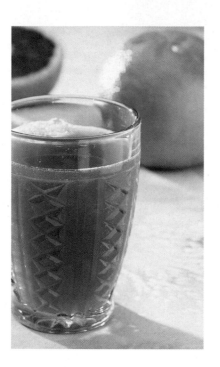

ELECTRIC VEGETABLE JUICERS

These devices turn solid pieces of vegetables and fruits into juices quickly and easily. Look for sturdy, well-constructed models from reputable manufacturers.

FOOD PROCESSORS AND BLENDERS

Both food processors and blenders are electrical devices designed to puree food. Food processors also come with blades designed for slicing and shredding. Look for sturdy models with good motors.

POTATO MASHER

This device has a long handle and flattened base to mash cooked potatoes. The base, usually made of metal, is either bent into parallel U shapes or else made with many holes. The potatoes are crushed by the base and broken into a thick, fluffy mass. Another device used to make mashed potatoes is a potato ricer. A pushing section forces potatoes through small holes in the bottom of the ricer.

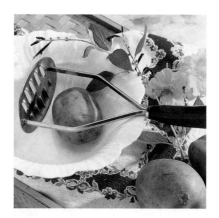

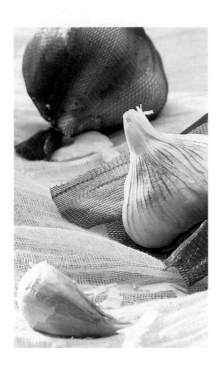

GARLIC PRESS

There are several styles of garlic presses available, but a good press should allow the user to force the garlic through the holes without much trouble. It should fit comfortably in the hand and clean without too much effort. You may want to look for a brand that comes with a reverse grid to press any remaining garlic out of the holes to aid in cleaning. In addition, you want to choose a press that is designed with an ergonomic grip. It may take some experimentation to find the press that works best for you.

VEGETABLE PEELER

This small tool becomes a lifesaver when you are faced with a mountain of potatoes for Thanksgiving, but will be appreciated for small jobs too. There are different styles available. Some models have the blade running in a straight line from the handle, others position the blade perpendicularly. The better styles have a swivel blade that compensates for the irregular surface of the vegetable being peeled. Some come with ergonomic grips. Experiment to find out which one suits you best. Discard peelers that have grown dull.

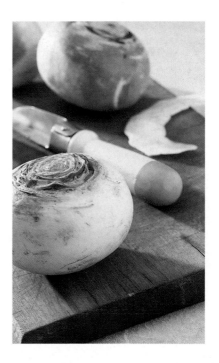

KNIVES

What makes a good knife? The best knives are often made of a combination of stainless and carbon steel, allowing for ease in sharpening while eliminating rust. Good knives have a piece of metal (called the tang) that extends from the blade down the length of the handle. This tang is attached by rivets. There are a variety of knives available to perform specific cutting tasks, but the knife best suited for such things as slicing, dicing and chopping is a chef's knife.

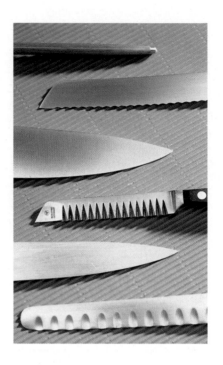

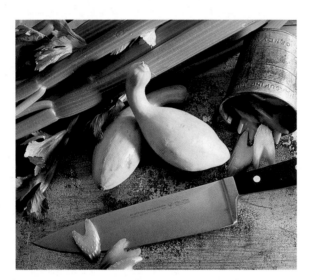

This chef's knife is extremely useful for slicing and chopping because of its elongated, triangular shape. Chef's knives come in several lengths; try to decide which length will be most comfortable for you and, if possible, see how it feels in your hand before purchase. Another useful knife is a small paring knife. It is very efficient for peeling, paring and other cutting jobs that involve smaller pieces of food. Asian chefs prefer using a cleaver, a hatchet-shaped knife that easily cuts through vegetables and meats.

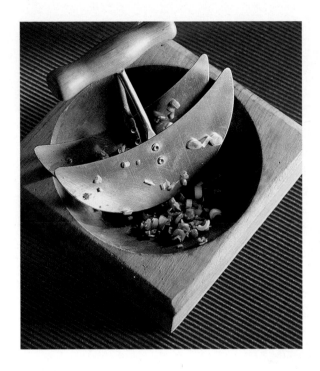

Italian cooks sometimes use a mezzaluna, a curved blade with handles on both ends. The blade chops and minces by rocking back and forth over food on a cutting board or in a rounded bowl.

MANDOLINES AND SLICERS

Mandolines are hand-operated, nonelectrical devices used for slicing and cutting vegetables into various sized strips. These tools have adjustable blades to allow for slicing and cutting in different thicknesses. The classic French mandoline is metal, but there are various plastic models available, some of which also shred and grate. An older American variation on this idea is the Feemster slicer, a simple device used for slicing. Protective guards

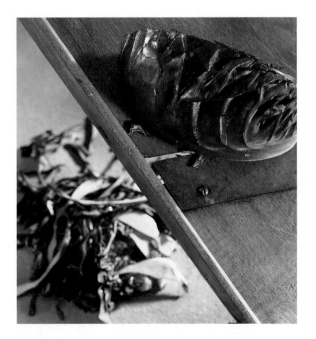

should be used to prevent cutting yourself. If protective guards aren't available, wear an oven mitt on the hand gripping the food you are slicing.

POTS AND PANS

Good quality pots and pans should be relatively heavy and conduct heat evenly. Certain metals — such as aluminum, copper and cast iron — conduct heat better than others. All of these metals can react with foods and are often sold with coatings or sealed in some way. Aluminum and cast iron can cause off-flavors or discoloration when used with certain foods, and copper generally needs to be lined with another metal for food safety reasons. Therefore, aluminum often comes sealed with a protective surface or combined in some way with stainless steel. Stainless steel is, by itself, a poor heat conductor and is usually combined with another metal. It contributes durability and does not react with foods. Cast iron is sometimes coated with enamel. Whether or not to use nonstick surfaces is another consideration. Food tends to brown better in a regular skillet, but nonstick aids significantly in cleanup.

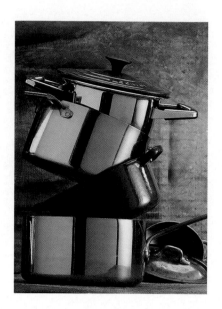

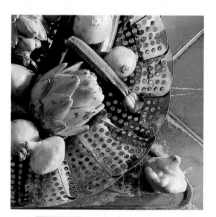

STEAMER INSERTS

The insert is placed inside a large pot that contains a small amount of water; the base has legs that keep the bottom out of the water. The collapsible side panels are expanded to form a basket, and vegetables are added. The water is brought to a boil and the pot is covered. The vegetables are steamed through holes in the bottom and sides of the insert. These inserts come in smaller and larger sizes to fit a variety of pots and pans.

$\mathcal{T}$IPS FOR TASTE

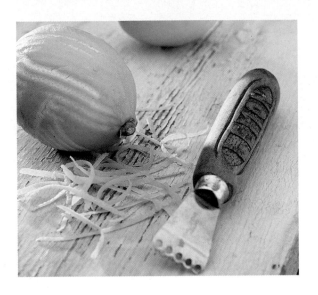

TIPS FOR TASTE

To jazz up vegetable side dishes, herbs are a great addition. Basil, dill, tarragon, thyme and many others go well with many vegetables.

Citrus is another easy flavor booster. A splash of lemon or a bit of orange or lime zest makes a dish taste fabulous with no effort.

Spicy seasonings add lots of zing too.

Nuts add crunch, and butter or olive oil makes everything taste better.

Sprinkle a bit of crumbled bacon or cheese over vegetables for another flavor boost.

Bottled sauces and spice blends can add flavor and zest to simple vegetable dishes when time is short.

Try different ethnic seasonings such as Thai or Indian for a change of pace.

Substitute different vegetables for the ones called for in recipes. Go ahead! For instance, if you don't have asparagus, try broccoli in the *Sesame Asparagus* (page 90) recipe.

Cooking is a creative process. Let your imagination and seasonal availability guide you to make cooking more pleasurable and eating a delight.

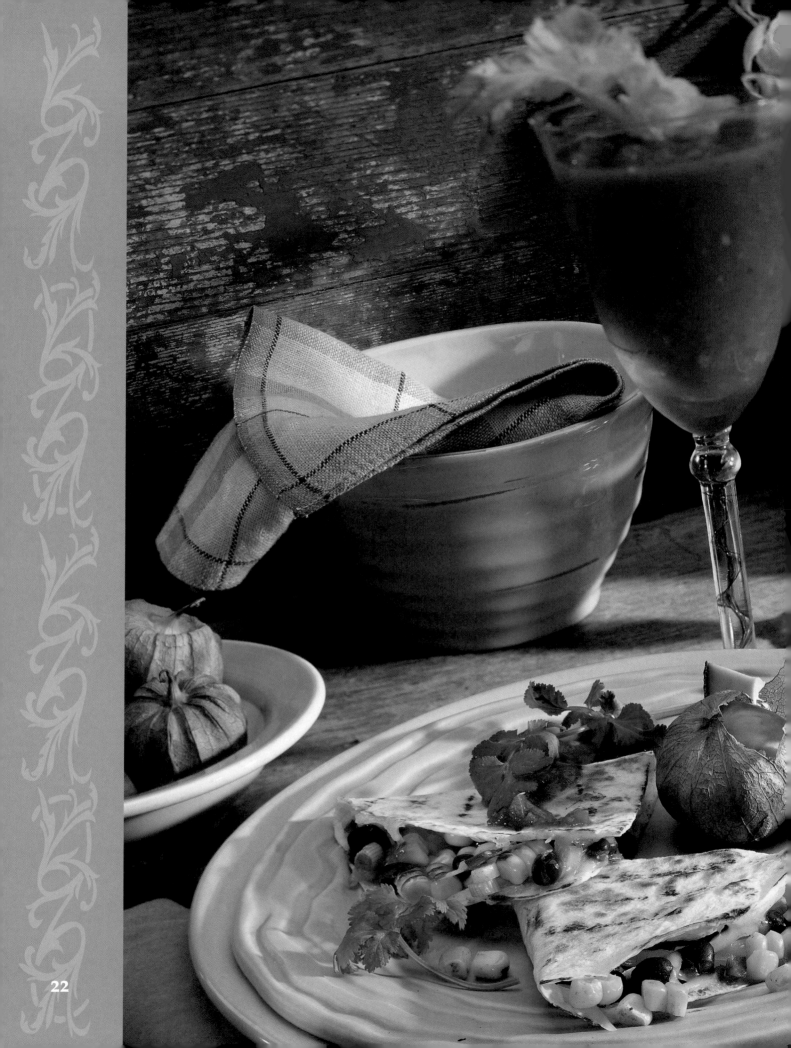

BEVERAGES & APPETIZERS

Try the two tempting juice recipes here as beverage options the next time you are entertaining. Along with the versatile selection of appetizers, they're a guaranteed hit. From easy to elegant, these thirst-quenchers and nibblers present plenty of afternoon pick-me-up options too.

Frosty Mary, page 24
Black Bean, Corn and Green Chile Quesadillas, page 25

FROSTY MARY

If a juicer is unavailable, use 1 quart of a purchased tomato-based vegetable juice. Freeze 2 cups with vodka and seasonings, omitting salt, and stir the slush mixture into the remaining 2 cups of juice the next day.

4	medium tomatoes
8	medium carrots
4	large ribs celery
1/2	cup vodka
1	teaspoon salt
1/4	teaspoon freshly ground pepper
1/4	teaspoon hot pepper sauce
1/4	teaspoon grated horseradish, if desired

1 The day before serving, juice 2 tomatoes, 4 carrots and 2 ribs celery in an electric vegetable juicer according to manufacturer's directions. Place in plastic container along with vodka, salt, pepper, hot pepper sauce and horseradish. Stir to combine. Freeze overnight, covered.

2 When ready to serve, juice remaining tomatoes, carrots and celery. Using tines of fork, break up frozen mixture into icy shreds; stir into juice or pulse in blender to combine. Divide evenly among 4 glasses. Garnish with celery, if desired. To make a nonalcoholic variation, simply omit the vodka. Do not freeze, but serve as juice.

4 servings.
Preparation time: 15 minutes. Ready to serve: 8 hours, 15 minutes.
Per serving: 165 calories, 1 g total fat (0 g saturated fat), 0 mg cholesterol, 700 mg sodium, 1.5 g fiber.

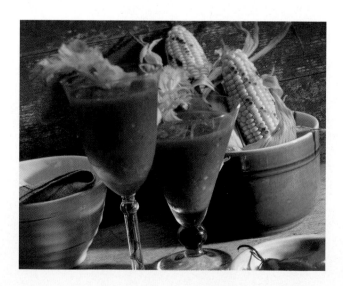

BLACK BEAN, CORN AND GREEN CHILE QUESADILLAS

Serve these quesadillas while relaxing on your patio on a perfect summer evening. If using a skillet on the grill to finish the quesadillas, make sure the handle is heat-resistant. Otherwise, finish them on the cooktop inside.

2	medium ears corn
2	Anaheim or New Mexico chiles
1	(15-oz.) can black beans, rinsed, drained
1/4	cup thinly sliced green onions
1	red jalapeño pepper, seeded, minced
1	tablespoon lime juice
1/2	teaspoon salt
4	(10-inch) flour tortillas
2	cups (8 oz.) shredded Monterey Jack cheese

❶ Remove silk from corn, leaving husks intact. Place corn and chiles on gas grill over medium-high heat or on charcoal grill 4 to 6 inches from medium-high coals. Grill chiles 8 to 10 minutes, turning when first side is charred. Grill corn about 12 minutes, turning 1/4 turn every 3 minutes.

❷ Remove chiles from heat; place in paper bag 5 minutes to loosen blackened skin. Remove corn from heat; let cool. Husk; remove kernels from cob. Place in medium bowl. Scrape skin from chiles; remove seeds and inner membranes. Chop chiles and place in bowl.

❸ Add black beans, onions, jalapeño, lime juice and salt. Divide mixture evenly among tortillas; spread on one half of each tortilla. Sprinkle each filled half with 1/2 cup of the cheese. Fold tortilla over filling.

❹ Heat large skillet or griddle on gas grill over medium-high heat or on charcoal grill 4 to 6 inches from medium-high coals, or on stove over medium-high heat. Cook each tortilla 4 minutes per side or until browned, turning once. Cut into quarters; serve with salsa, if desired.

8 servings.
Preparation time: 15 minutes. Ready to serve: 47 minutes.
Per serving: 290 calories, 11.5 g total fat (6 g saturated fat), 25 mg cholesterol, 570 mg sodium, 4.5 g fiber.

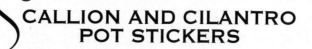

SCALLION AND CILANTRO POT STICKERS

Look for wonton skins in the produce or Asian section of large supermarkets, or in specialty food stores.

4	tablespoons vegetable oil
1	tablespoon chopped fresh ginger
1	cup chopped green onions, including tender green portion of stem
2½	cups chopped Savoy or Napa cabbage
2	tablespoons soy sauce
⅓	cup chopped cilantro
1½	teaspoons toasted sesame oil
24	wonton skins
⅔	cup water

❶ Heat 2 tablespoons of the vegetable oil in large nonstick skillet over high heat until hot. Add ginger; sauté 30 to 60 seconds or until fragrant. Add onions; sauté 2 to 3 minutes to soften slightly. Add cabbage and soy sauce; sauté 3 to 4 minutes or until cabbage is wilted and most of moisture is evaporated. Remove from heat; stir in cilantro and sesame oil. Place in medium bowl; cool.

❷ In center of each skin, place heaping teaspoonful of cabbage mixture. Moisten edges of skin with water. Fold skin in half to form half-moon shape. Pinch and pleat top layer of skin along rounded edge. Press edges of skin together to seal.

❸ Heat 1 tablespoon of the vegetable oil in large nonstick skillet over high heat until hot. Reduce heat to medium-high; add half of pot stickers, unfluted side down. Cook 2 to 3 minutes or until lightly browned on bottom. Add ⅓ cup of the water; cover and steam 3 to 4 minutes. Remove cover; cook an additional 1 to 2 minutes or until pot stickers are deep brown on bottom. Remove from skillet and repeat process, using remaining 1 tablespoon vegetable oil and ⅓ cup water to cook second half of pot stickers. Serve with citrus-soy dipping sauce.*

TIP *To make citrus-soy dipping sauce, see recipe for *Spring Rolls* (page 31).

24 pot stickers.
Preparation time: 40 minutes. Ready to serve: 52 minutes.

Per sticker: 60 calories, 4 g total fat (.5 g saturated fat), 5 mg cholesterol, 265 mg sodium, .5 g fiber.

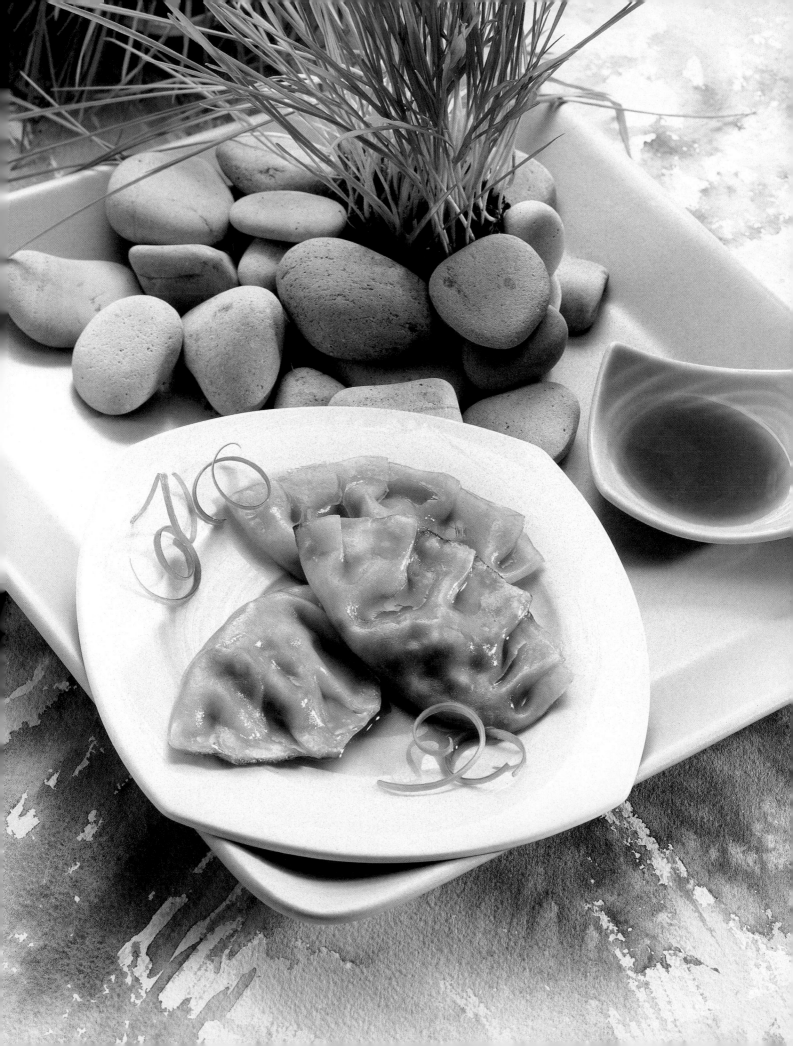

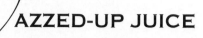

JAZZED-UP JUICE

Try this peppy juice for a healthy, thirst-quenching beverage. If you don't have a juicer, combine 2/3 cup canned carrot juice with 1/3 cup apple juice for a tasty introduction to what juicing is all about.

4　medium carrots
2　large ribs celery
1　jalapeño pepper, seeded

❶ In electric vegetable juicer, process carrots, celery and jalapeño according to manufacturer's directions.

2½ servings.
Preparation time: 5 minutes. Ready to serve: 5 minutes.

Per serving: 65 calories, .5 g total fat (0 g saturated fat), 0 mg cholesterol, 85 mg sodium, 1 g fiber.

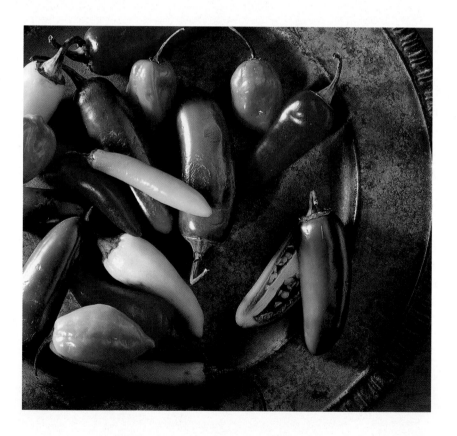

GREAT GARLICKY DIP WITH SUMMER VEGETABLES

Roasted garlic is much milder than raw, and it is a perfect complement to the beans and olive oil in this flavorful dip. Try using the dip as a spread for sandwiches too.

- 1 large head garlic
- 2 tablespoons plus 1/2 teaspoon extra-virgin olive oil
- 1 tablespoon water
- 1 (15-oz.) can cannellini beans, rinsed, drained
- 1 tablespoon lemon juice
- 1/2 teaspoon salt
  Dash ground red pepper
- 6 cups assorted summer vegetables (cherry tomatoes, blanched green beans, zucchini spears, baby carrots, pattypan squash) cut into pieces

1. Heat oven to 350°F. Remove outer papery skin of garlic. Cut pointed top of garlic to expose flesh. Place in center of 12-inch square piece of foil; drizzle with 1/2 teaspoon of the olive oil. Pull up edges of foil to form pouch; add water. Tighten edge of foil to seal; place in oven. Bake about 1 hour or until garlic is soft. Remove; let cool.

2. Squeeze flesh of garlic from skin into bowl of food processor. Add beans; pulse to puree. Add remaining 2 tablespoons oil, lemon juice, salt and red pepper; pulse to combine. Place in small bowl; cover and refrigerate several hours to infuse flavors. Serve with vegetables.

12 servings.
Preparation time: 15 minutes. Ready to serve: 4 hours, 5 minutes.

Per serving: 75 calories, 2.5 g total fat (.5 g saturated fat), 0 mg cholesterol, 165 mg sodium, 3.5 g fiber.

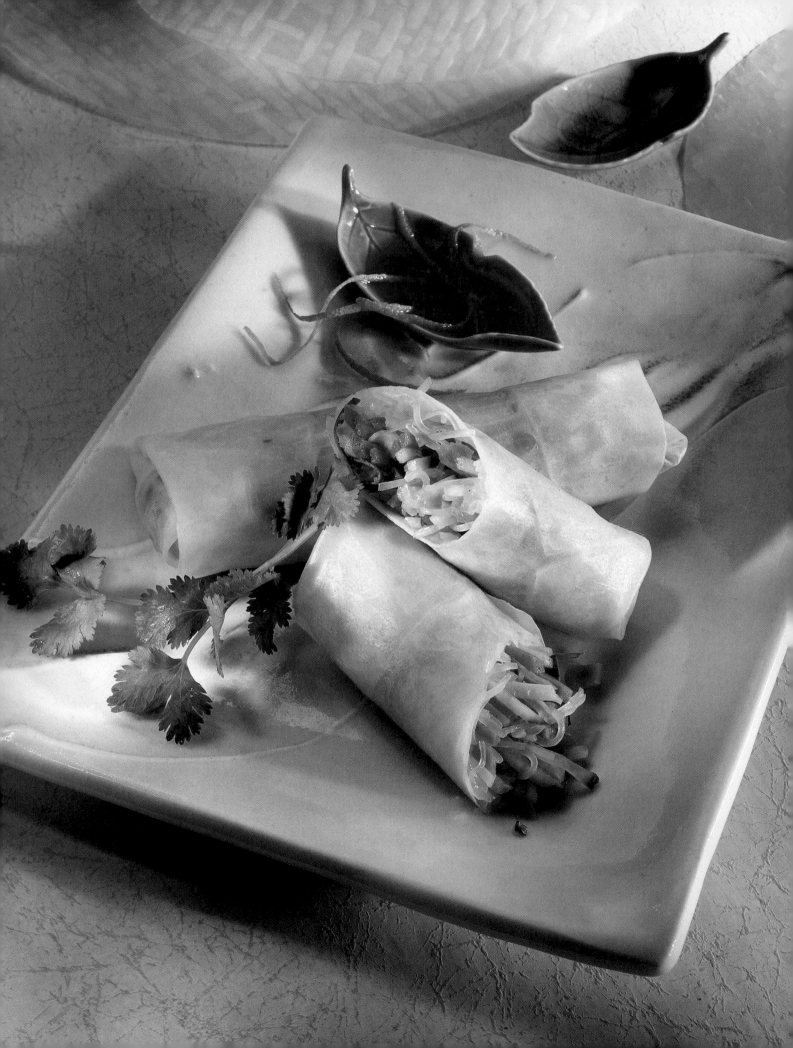

SPRING ROLLS

Unlike fried spring rolls, these fresh rolls let the true flavor of the ingredients shine through. Look for the wrappers, sometimes called rice paper wrappers, in Asian markets or in large supermarkets.

FILLING

1   oz. bean thread noodles
1   cup shredded carrots
1/2   cup matchstick-size strips cucumber
1/2   cup whole fresh cilantro
1/4   cup slivered green onions
1/4   cup shredded turnip
1/4   cup chopped peanuts
2   tablespoons coarsely chopped fresh basil
2   tablespoons coarsely chopped fresh mint
1/2   jalapeño pepper, slivered
1/4   teaspoon salt
8   dried spring roll wrappers

DIPPING SAUCE

1/4   cup soy sauce
1/4   cup orange juice
1/4   cup water
2   tablespoons white or red wine vinegar
2   tablespoons slivered green onion
1   teaspoon grated orange peel

❶ Place noodles in medium bowl; cover with boiling water. Soak 15 minutes. Drain; cut into 1-inch pieces.

❷ In large bowl, combine noodles, carrots, cucumber, cilantro, onion, turnip, peanuts, basil, mint, jalapeño and salt. In shallow dish, soak each wrapper in hot water until soft. Drain on towel. Place 1/8 of mixture on lower edge of each wrapper. Shape into tight cylinder by folding curved bottom edge up and over to enclose filling in one tight turn. Fold both outside edges inward to enclose filling at both ends. Continue rolling into packed cylinder. Cut in half diagonally.

❸ In small bowl, combine soy sauce, orange juice, water, vinegar, green onion and grated peel. Serve with Spring Rolls.

8 servings. Preparation time: 30 minutes. Ready to serve: 30 minutes.

Per serving: 80 calories, 2.5 g total fat (.5 g saturated fat), 5 mg cholesterol, 600 mg sodium, 1.5 g fiber.

SPINACH PESTO-STUFFED MUSHROOMS

The bread crumbs in the mixture absorb excess moisture from the spinach and mushrooms. To cut back on oil, try spraying the mushroom caps with olive oil-flavored nonstick cooking spray instead of brushing them with olive oil.

- 1 large garlic clove
- 2 cups coarsely chopped fresh spinach
- 1/2 cup coarsely chopped fresh basil
- 1/3 cup dry bread crumbs
- 1/4 cup (1 oz.) freshly grated Parmesan cheese
- 5 tablespoons extra-virgin olive oil
- 1 lb. medium mushrooms (32 to 36 mushrooms), stems removed

❶ Heat oven to 400°F. With motor running, drop garlic clove into bowl of food processor to chop. Add spinach and basil; pulse until very finely chopped. Add bread crumbs and cheese; pulse to combine. With motor running, add 3 tablespoons of the oil to form thick paste.

❷ Brush mushroom caps with remaining 2 tablespoons oil; place on shallow baking sheet. Fill each cap with about 1 teaspoon filling, pressing into cavity and mounding on top. Bake 15 to 20 minutes or until mushrooms are tender and filling is hot.

32 to 36 mushrooms.
Preparation time: 15 minutes. Ready to serve: 30 minutes.

Per mushroom: 30 calories, 2.5 g total fat (.5 g saturated fat), 0 mg cholesterol, 30 mg sodium, .5 g fiber.

SOUTHWESTERN ROASTED PUMPKIN SEEDS

Raw pepitas are pumpkin seeds used in Mexican cooking. They can be found in health food stores, supermarkets or Hispanic grocery stores. If unavailable, substitute your favorite raw nut.

2   tablespoons vegetable oil
1   tablespoon chili powder
1   teaspoon cider vinegar
1   teaspoon garlic salt
1/2   teaspoon ground cumin
1/2   teaspoon cayenne
1/4   teaspoon salt
2   cups raw pepitas

❶ Heat oven to 350°F. In medium bowl, combine oil, chili powder, vinegar, garlic salt, cumin, cayenne and salt. Stir to combine. Add pepitas; stir to coat. Spread on 15x10x1-inch pan. Bake 10 to 15 minutes, or until browned and crisp, stirring every 5 minutes. Remove from oven; cool. Scrape pepitas and seasonings into bowl; stir briefly.

8 servings.
Preparation time: 5 minutes. Ready to serve: 15 minutes.

Per serving: 215 calories, 18 g total fat (3.5 g saturated fat), 0 mg cholesterol, 210 mg sodium, 2.5 g fiber.

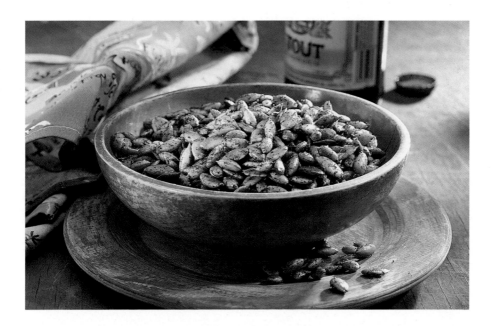

TEX-MEX POTATO SKINS

These spicy appetizers are perfect while watching a football game or for casual entertaining. The pepper Jack cheese adds extra heat. If not available, seed and chop two jalapeño peppers and sprinkle over 4 ounces of Monterey Jack cheese.

4	medium-large russet potatoes
1/2	teaspoon garlic salt
2	oz. shredded cheddar cheese
2	oz. shredded pepper Jack cheese
1/2	cup sour cream
1	cup medium-chunky salsa
1/2	cup sliced green onion tops

❶ Heat oven to 400°F. Prick potatoes in several places with fork or tip of knife; bake on baking sheet at 400°F for about 1 1/4 to 1 1/2 hours, or until slightly overdone (skins should be crispy and firm). Let cool on wire rack; cut into quarters. With spoon, remove most of flesh. Reduce oven temperature to 350°F.

❷ Line 2 baking sheets with aluminum foil or parchment paper. Place potato skins on baking sheets, flesh side up. Sprinkle lightly with salt. In medium bowl, combine cheddar and pepper Jack cheese; top each potato skin with 2 tablespoons cheese mixture. Bake potato skins at 350°F for 5 to 8 minutes or until cheese is melted.

❸ Top each potato skin with 1 tablespoon of the sour cream; drizzle each with salsa. Sprinkle with onions.

8 servings.
Preparation time: 10 minutes. Ready to serve: 1 hour, 30 minutes.
Per serving: 145 calories, 7.5 g total fat (4.5 g saturated fat), 25 mg cholesterol, 240 mg sodium, 1.5 g fiber.

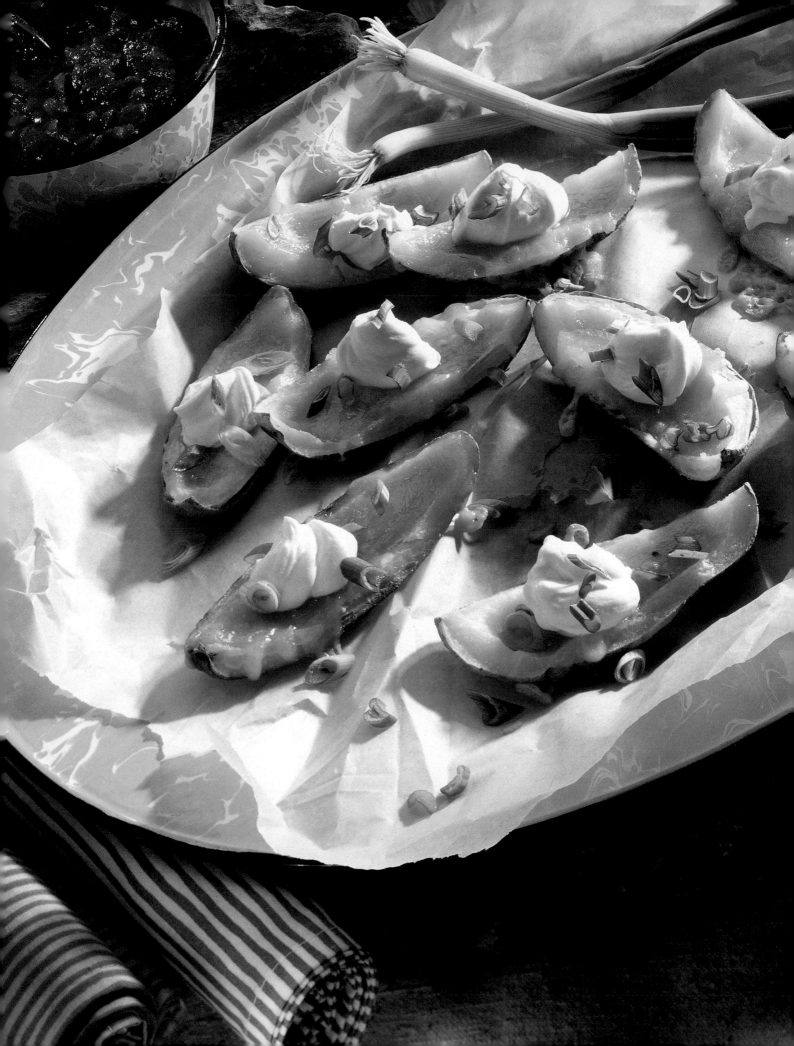

VEGETARIAN FONDUE

Double this recipe and use it as a relaxing main course. Emmentaler cheese is the real thing — cheese from Switzerland with holes throughout. You may substitute Swiss Gruyère or another high-quality imported Swiss-style cheese.

  1 tablespoon cornstarch
1/4 teaspoon dry ground mustard
  1 cup plus 2 tablespoons white wine
  1 whole clove garlic, peeled, slightly crushed
12 oz. Emmentaler cheese, cut into 1/4-inch cubes
     Dash ground nutmeg
     Hearty rye bread loaf, cut into 1-inch cubes
     Vegetables of your choice

❶ In small bowl, combine cornstarch and dry mustard; mix well. Add 2 tablespoons wine; stir to combine. Set aside.

❷ Heat 1 cup wine and garlic in medium saucepan over low heat until bubbles begin to appear around edges of wine. Remove garlic. Add cheese and nutmeg; stir until cheese begins to melt. Stir in cornstarch mixture; continue to cook about 5 minutes or until mixture begins to thicken, stirring constantly. Pour into fondue pot or heat-proof serving dish; set over flame. Serve with bread, and your choice of broccoli, cauliflower and eggplant.

8 servings.
Preparation time: 15 minutes. Ready to serve: 20 minutes.

Per serving: 200 calories, 12 g total fat (7.5 g saturated fat), 40 mg cholesterol, 175 mg sodium, 1.5 g fiber.

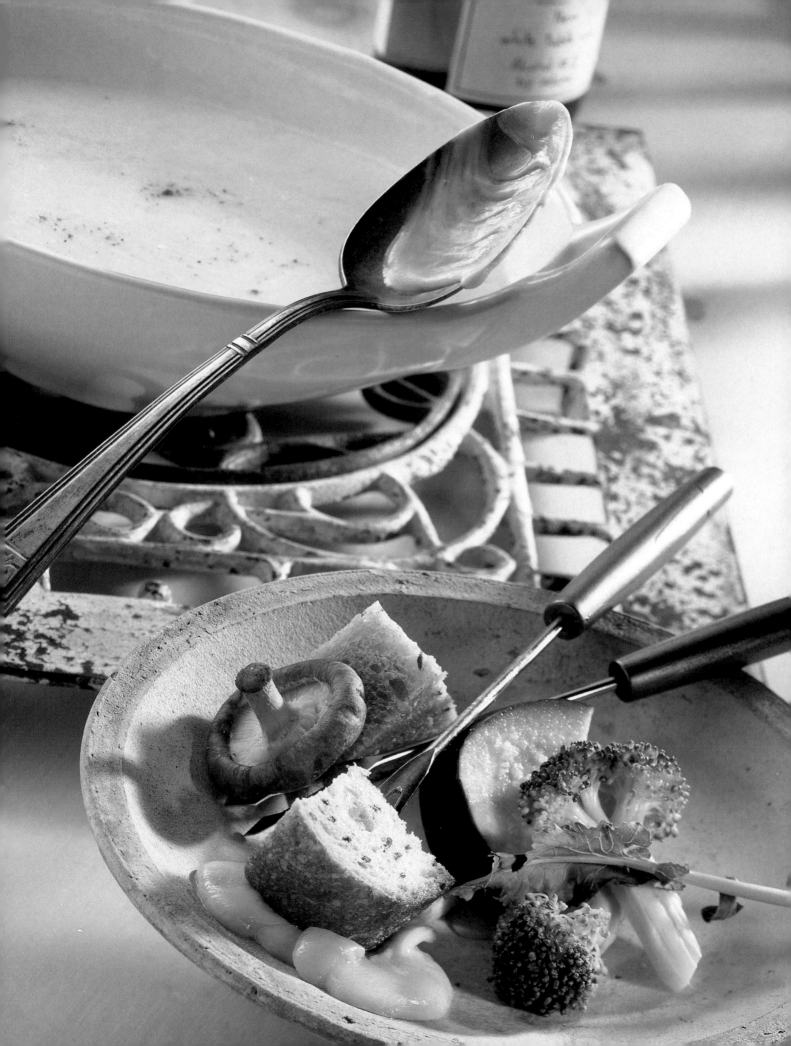

CARAMELIZED ONION AND GOAT CHEESE PHYLLO TRIANGLES

Look for phyllo dough in the freezer section of the grocery store. Before using, thaw in the refrigerator 6 to 8 hours or overnight. While working with one sheet, cover the others with a barely dampened towel to keep them from drying out. Wrap unused phyllo tightly and refreeze for later use.

- 2 tablespoons vegetable oil
- 2 medium onions, thinly sliced
- 1/2 teaspoon sugar
- 1/2 teaspoon dried thyme
- 1/4 teaspoon salt
- 1/8 teaspoon freshly ground pepper
- 1 (3.5- to 4-oz.) package goat cheese
- 4 (14 x 18-inch) sheets frozen phyllo, thawed
- 5 tablespoons butter, melted

① Heat oil in large skillet over medium heat until hot. Add onions; sauté onions about 5 minutes, or until slightly softened, stirring occasionally. Reduce heat to low; cover and cook 5 minutes, stirring occasionally. Uncover; add sugar. Cook an additional 10 to 15 minutes or until onions are very soft and golden brown. Add thyme, salt and pepper; mix well. Remove from heat. Let cool. Stir in goat cheese.

② Heat oven to 400°F. Place 1 sheet of phyllo on cutting board; brush with butter. Cut into 8 (2¼ x 14-inch) strips. Place 1 teaspoon goat cheese mixture in lower right corner of each strip. Fold corners up and over to enclose filling, forming a triangle. Continue each strip and fold one corner to opposite side to form triangle. Continue to fold, triangle fashion, up length of strip. Brush with melted butter; place on ungreased baking sheet. Repeat with remaining strips, and remaining 3 sheets phyllo.

③ Bake 10 to 12 minutes or until phyllo triangles are browned and crisp. Serve warm or room temperature.

32 triangles. Preparation time: 50 minutes. Ready to serve: 1 hour.

Per triangle: 48 calories, 4 g total fat (2 g saturated fat), 10 mg cholesterol, 50 mg sodium, 0 g fiber.

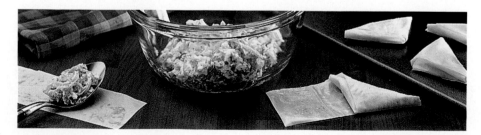

SPRING SUGAR SNAPS, ASPARAGUS SPEARS AND RADISHES WITH MINT-CHIVE DIP

This recipe uses spring's wonderful produce and herbs to make a delightful hors d'oeuvre. To prepare asparagus, hold the spear with two hands, bend slightly and snap off the unyielding portion at the end. If the skin seems tough, remove with a vegetable peeler. Submerge in water and swirl spears to remove any grit lodged in the tips.

3/4 lb. sugar snap peas
3/4 lb. asparagus spears, trimmed, cut into 2½-inch pieces
1/2 lb. radishes

DIP
1 cup sour cream
2 tablespoons chopped fresh mint
2 tablespoons chopped fresh chives
1/4 teaspoon salt
1/8 teaspoon freshly ground pepper

❶ Fill large saucepan half full with water. Bring to a boil over high heat; add peas and asparagus. Cook 2 minutes. Drain; run peas and asparagus under cold water to stop cooking. Cover; set aside until ready to serve.

❷ In small bowl, combine sour cream, mint, chives, salt and pepper. Serve with peas, asparagus and radishes.

8 servings.
Preparation time: 20 minutes. Ready to serve: 20 minutes.
Per serving: 90 calories, 6 g total fat (3.5 g saturated fat), 20 mg cholesterol, 95 mg sodium, 2.5 g fiber.

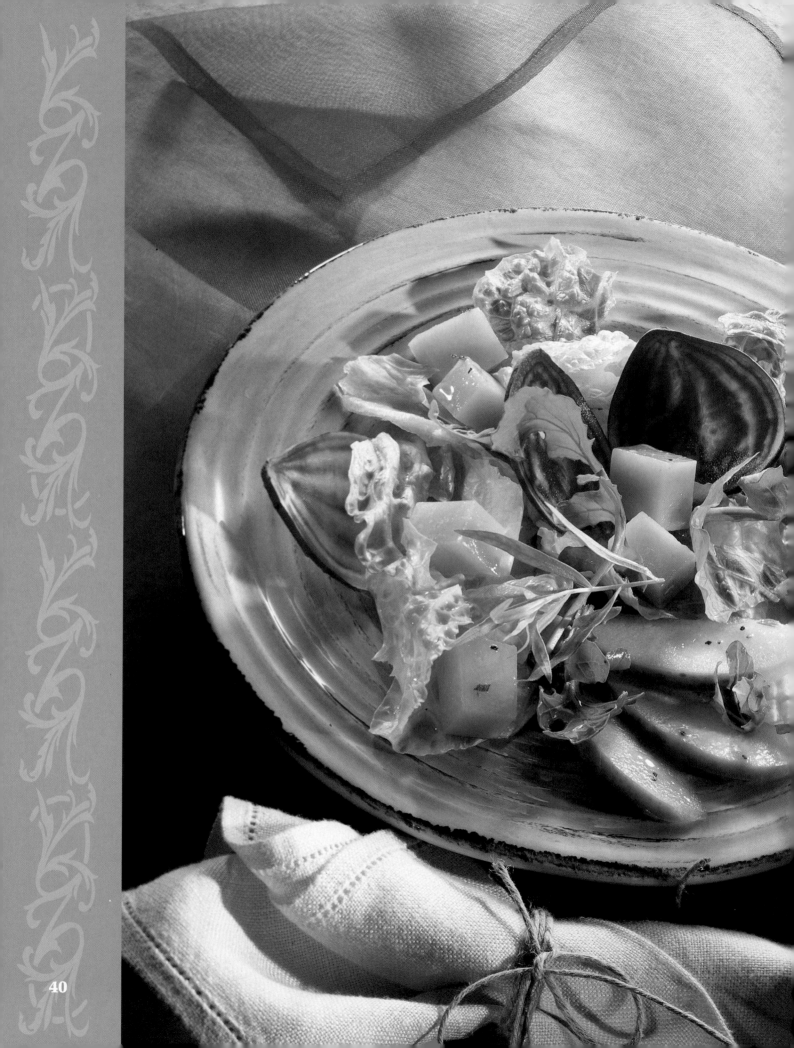

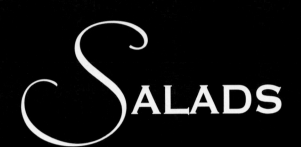

SALADS

There's something refreshingly satisfying about a salad. The cool crunch of crisp lettuce paired with tangy dressing brings taste buds alive with each bite. Versatile in nature, salads welcome a variety of produce plus such diverse additions as bread or grains. Make up your own combinations! And try different vinegars and oils for endless dressing possibilities.

Beet, Apple and Gruyère Salad, page 42

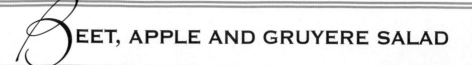

BEET, APPLE AND GRUYERE SALAD

If available, try substituting yellow or candy cane striped beets for the red variety. Make sure to add the beets first, before the apples or cheese, to keep their vivid colors separate from the other ingredients.

VINAIGRETTE

2 tablespoons cider vinegar

1½ teaspoons Dijon mustard

½ cup vegetable oil

1½ teaspoons chopped fresh tarragon or ½ teaspoon dried

⅛ teaspoon salt

Pinch freshly ground pepper

SALAD

1 large or 2 small cooked beets, peeled, thinly sliced*

1 large Granny Smith apple, thinly sliced

8 cups bite-size pieces romaine lettuce and arugula

4 oz. Gruyère cheese, cut into ½-inch pieces

❶ In small bowl, whisk together vinegar and mustard. Slowly whisk in oil. Whisk in tarragon, salt and pepper.

❷ Place beets in another small bowl; toss with generous tablespoon of vinaigrette. Place apple in separate small bowl; toss with another generous tablespoon of vinaigrette. Place salad greens in large bowl and toss with remaining vinaigrette. Divide greens evenly among 6 salad plates. Sprinkle greens evenly with beets, apples and cheese. Serve immediately.

TIP *To cook beets, trim tops to about 2 inches; leave root stem intact. Wash to remove dirt but do not peel until after cooking. Place in medium saucepan with enough water to cover. Add 1 teaspoon salt; boil over medium-high heat until tender, about 20 to 25 minutes for small beets, 35 to 40 for medium and 45 to 50 for large. If cooking a large amount of beets, increase pan size, water volume and salt accordingly.

6 servings.
Preparation time: 20 minutes. Ready to serve: 1 hour, 5 minutes.

Per serving: 270 calories, 23.5 g total fat (6 g saturated fat), 15 mg cholesterol, 125 mg sodium, 2.5 g fiber.

CORN AND BARLEY SALAD

Barley is a grain commonly used in soups and breads, but it makes a delicious addition to this main dish salad.

2/3 cup barley
2 cups cooked corn kernels
1 red bell pepper, cut into 1/2-inch pieces
1/4 cup chopped green onions
1/4 cup extra-virgin olive oil
2 teaspoons grated lime zest
2 tablespoons freshly squeezed lime juice
1 tablespoon chopped fresh cilantro
1/2 teaspoon ground cumin
1/2 teaspoon garlic salt
1/2 teaspoon salt
1/8 teaspoon hot pepper sauce

❶ Cook barley according to package directions. Let cool.

❷ In large bowl, combine barley, corn, bell pepper and onions. In small bowl, whisk together oil, lime zest, lime juice, cilantro, cumin, salts and hot pepper sauce. Pour over barley mixture; toss to coat. Chill several hours to allow flavors to blend.

4 main dish or 6 side dish servings.
Preparation time: 20 minutes. Ready to serve: 3 hours, 30 minutes.

Per main dish serving: 345 calories, 14.5 g total fat (2 g saturated fat), 0 mg cholesterol, 480 mg sodium, 9 g fiber.

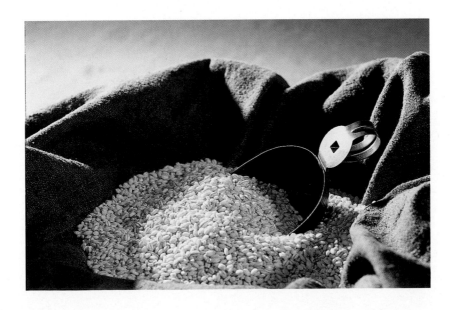

FRESH TOMATO SALAD WITH PESTO CROUTONS

Try these tasty croutons in your favorite tomato soup or with other summer salads.

CROUTONS
- 1/4 cup extra-virgin olive oil
- 1/4 cup lightly packed, coarsely chopped fresh basil leaves
- 2 tablespoons freshly grated Parmesan cheese
- 6 (3/4-inch) slices stale baguette, cut into 3/4-inch cubes

DRESSING
- 2 tablespoons extra-virgin olive oil
- 1 tablespoon lemon juice
- 1/4 teaspoon salt
- 1/8 teaspoon freshly ground pepper

SALAD
- 1/4 cup chopped red onion
- 4 cups torn leaf lettuce
- 3 medium red tomatoes, sliced
- 3 medium yellow tomatoes, sliced

1. Place 1/4 cup oil, basil and cheese in blender or food processor. Pulse to puree. Pour into medium bowl. Add bread; toss to coat. Heat large skillet over medium-high heat until hot. Add bread; cook 5 to 7 minutes or until brown and crispy, turning often. Set aside.

2. In small bowl whisk together oil, lemon juice, salt and pepper. Set aside.

3. Place onion in another small bowl; cover with cold water. Soak 15 minutes; drain well. Spread lettuce over serving platter. Top with overlapping rows of tomatoes, alternating colors and beginning with a row of red tomatoes. Repeat until all tomatoes are used. Sprinkle with onion; drizzle with dressing. Sprinkle with croutons.

6 servings.
Preparation time: 15 minutes. Ready to serve: 30 minutes.
Per serving: 200 calories, 15 g total fat (2.5 g saturated fat), 0 mg cholesterol, 235 mg sodium, 2.5 g fiber.

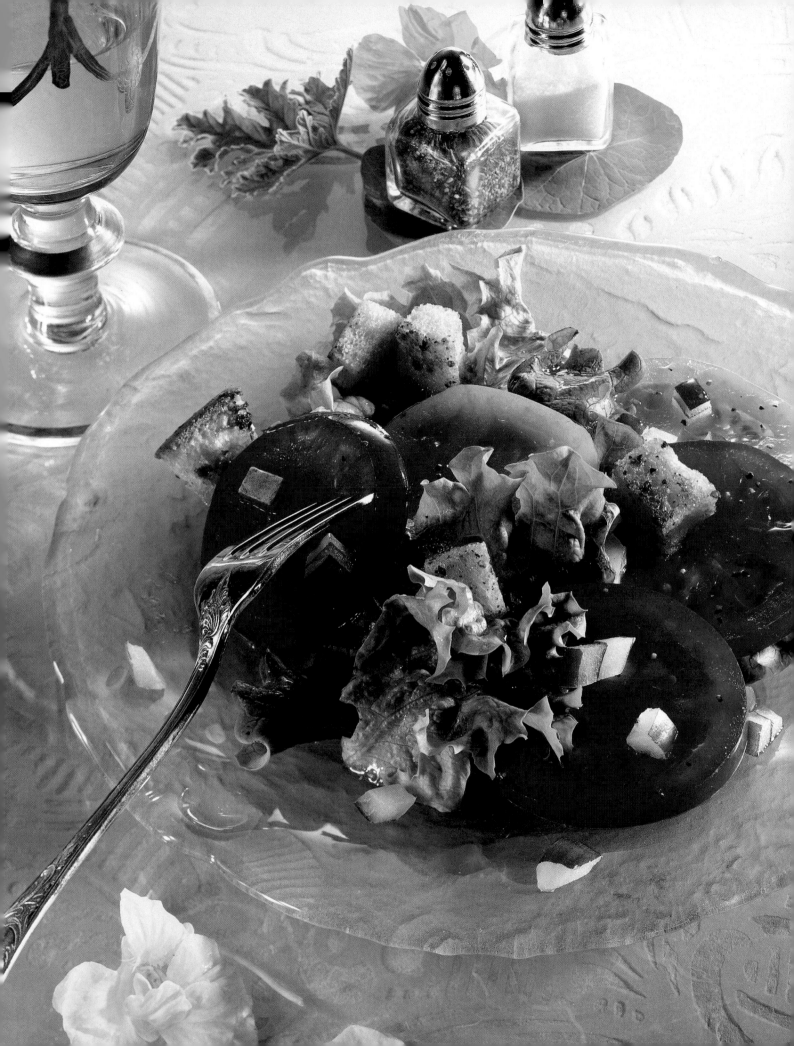

BREAD SALAD WITH GRILLED ZUCCHINI

This popular Italian salad is a great way to use up leftover French bread. Be sure to make it in the summer when tomatoes and basil are at their peak!

1   (8-oz.) slightly stale baguette
3   medium-small (about ³/4 lb.) zucchini, cut lengthwise
       into ¹/2-inch wide strips
1   small red onion, cut into ¹/2-inch wide slices
¹/2 cup plus 1 tablespoon extra-virgin olive oil
2   large tomatoes, cut into 1-inch pieces
¹/2 cup coarsely chopped fresh basil
¹/4 cup chopped fresh Italian parsley
¹/4 cup red wine vinegar
2   tablespoons water
1¹/2 teaspoons minced garlic
¹/2 teaspoon salt
¹/4 teaspoon freshly ground pepper
¹/4 cup (1 oz.) freshly grated Parmesan cheese

❶ Cut baguette into 1¹/2-inch pieces. Place on tray and allow to dry slightly while preparing remainder of salad.

❷ Heat grill. Brush zucchini and onion slices lightly with 1 tablespoon of the olive oil. Grill zucchini and onion on gas grill over medium heat or on charcoal grill 4 to 6 inches from medium coals 10 minutes, or until crisp tender, turning once. Remove; cool slightly. Cut into 1-inch pieces.

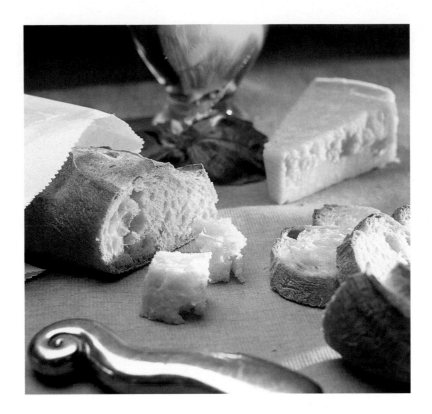

❸ In large bowl, combine bread, zucchini, onion, tomatoes, basil and parsley; toss to combine. In small bowl, whisk together remaining ½ cup oil, vinegar, water, garlic, salt and pepper. Drizzle dressing over salad, tossing to coat. Sprinkle with cheese.

8 servings.
Preparation time: 20 minutes. Ready to serve: 30 minutes.
Per serving: 255 calories, 17.5 g total fat (3 g saturated fat), 5 mg cholesterol, 385 mg sodium, 2.5 g fiber.

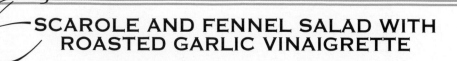

ESCAROLE AND FENNEL SALAD WITH ROASTED GARLIC VINAIGRETTE

Ideal in late fall and winter, escarole's bite is complemented by fennel's sweetness. Iceberg lettuce provides a crunchy background, while the roasted garlic vinaigrette pulls everything together.

VINAIGRETTE
- 1 head garlic, roasted*
- 1/3 cup extra-virgin olive oil
- 2 tablespoons red wine vinegar
- 1/2 teaspoon Dijon mustard
- 1/4 teaspoon salt
- 1/8 teaspoon freshly ground pepper

SALAD
- 4 cups bite-size pieces escarole
- 4 cups bite-size pieces iceberg lettuce
- 1 medium fennel bulb, fronds removed, quartered, cut into 1/4-inch slices

❶ In blender, combine roasted garlic, oil, vinegar, mustard, salt and pepper. Puree until creamy and well blended.

❷ Just before serving, toss escarole, lettuce and fennel bulb with vinaigrette.

TIP *To roast garlic, see directions in recipe for *Great Garlicky Dip with Summer Vegetables* (page 29).

6 servings.
Preparation time: 15 minutes. Ready to serve: 1 hour, 15 minutes.
Per serving: 135 calories, 12 g total fat (1.5 g saturated fat), 0 mg cholesterol, 130 mg sodium, 2 g fiber.

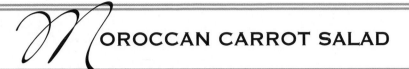

MOROCCAN CARROT SALAD

Inspired by North African flavors, this salad will quickly become a family favorite.

- 2 tablespoons lemon juice
- 1 tablespoon orange juice
- 1 tablespoon honey
- 1/2 teaspoon ground cumin
- 1/2 teaspoon salt
- 1/4 teaspoon cinnamon
- 4 large carrots, grated (about 3 cups)

❶ Combine lemon juice, orange juice, honey, cumin, salt and cinnamon in medium bowl; mix well. Add carrots; toss to combine. (Carrots will lose volume when dressed.)

4 servings.
Preparation time: 15 minutes. Ready to serve: 15 minutes.

Per serving: 70 calories, .5 g total fat (0 g saturated fat), 0 mg cholesterol, 330 mg sodium, 3.5 g fiber.

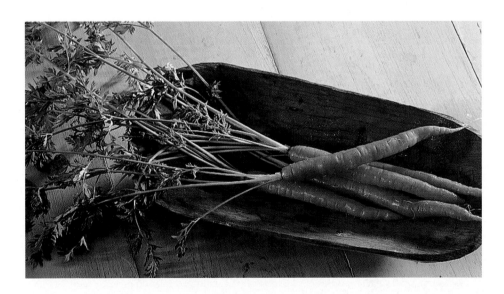

*I*TALIAN WHEAT BERRY SALAD

Wheat berries are whole kernels of wheat. Look for them in natural food stores. If unavailable, substitute cracked wheat or bulgur, cooked according to package directions.

- 1 cup wheat berries
- 2 teaspoons salt
- 1 yellow bell pepper, cut into 1/2-inch pieces
- 1 medium carrot, cut into 1/2-inch pieces
- 12 cherry tomatoes, halved
- 1 small zucchini, cut into 1/2-inch pieces
- 1/3 cup chopped fresh basil
- 1/4 cup finely sliced green onions
- 1 (6.5-oz.) jar marinated artichoke hearts
- 6 tablespoons extra-virgin olive oil
- 3 tablespoons balsamic vinegar
- 1 teaspoon finely minced garlic
- 1 1/2 teaspoons chopped fresh rosemary or 1/2 teaspoon dried rosemary, crushed
- 1/8 teaspoon freshly ground pepper

1 Place wheat berries in medium saucepan with enough water to cover by several inches. Cook over low heat 2 hours or until tender, adding 1 1/2 teaspoons of the salt during last 30 minutes of cooking. Drain; cool.

2 In large bowl, combine wheat berries with bell pepper, carrot, tomatoes, zucchini, basil and onions. Drain artichokes, reserving marinade. Cut artichokes into 1/2-inch pieces; add to wheat berry mixture.

3 In small bowl, combine reserved marinade, oil, vinegar, garlic, rosemary, salt and pepper; mix well. Toss with wheat berry mixture. Chill several hours to allow flavors to blend.

4 main course or 6 side dish servings.
Preparation time: 15 minutes. Ready to serve: 5 hours, 15 minutes.

Per main course serving: 350 calories, 22.5 g total fat (3 g saturated fat), 0 mg cholesterol, 740 mg sodium, 8 g fiber.

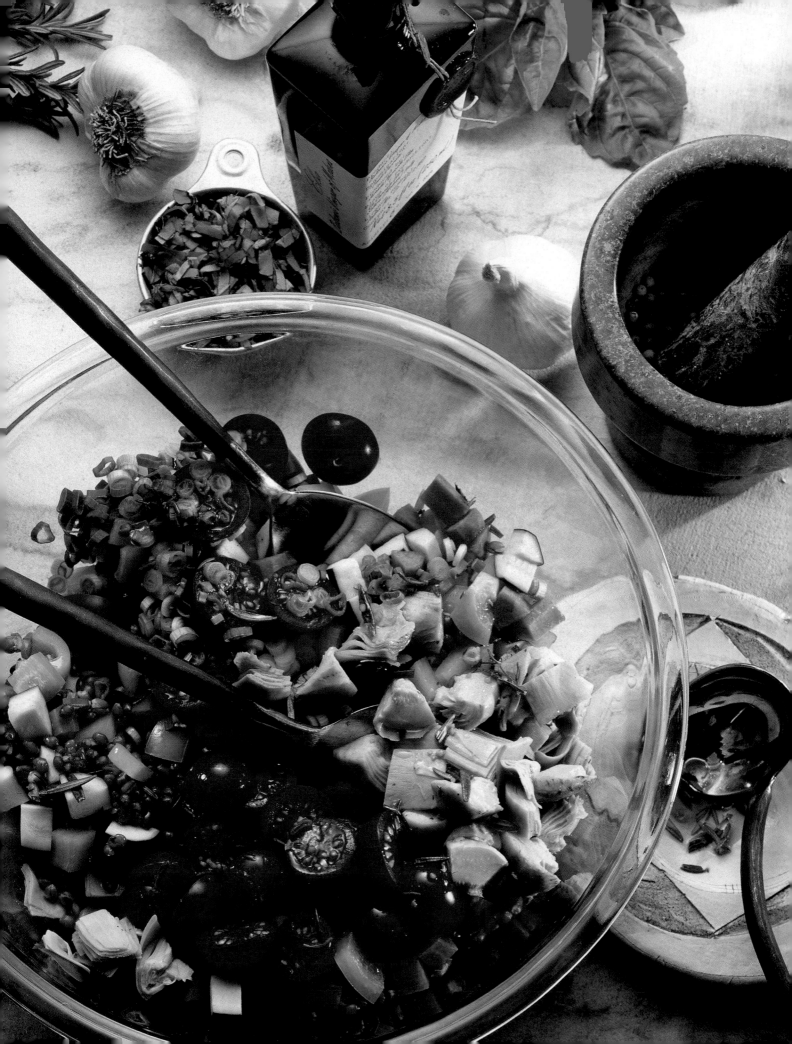

GAZPACHO SALAD WITH SPICED CORN CROUTONS

Use leftover cornbread to make these tasty croutons, or feel free to substitute your favorite purchased croutons if time is of the essence.

CROUTONS

- 1½ cups cubed (¾ inch) stale cornbread
- ½ teaspoon chili powder
- ¼ teaspoon garlic salt
- Dash cayenne

SALAD

- 1 large tomato
- 1 medium cucumber, peeled
- 1 small to medium green bell pepper, seeded
- 3 green onions
- 6 cups torn leaf lettuce

DRESSING

- 5 tablespoons extra-virgin olive oil
- 1 tablespoon sherry vinegar or red wine vinegar
- 1 teaspoon minced garlic
- ⅛ teaspoon salt
- Dash cayenne

1. Heat oven to 350°F. Place cornbread in shallow baking pan; spray with nonstick cooking spray. In small bowl, combine chili powder, garlic salt and cayenne; sprinkle over cornbread. Bake 10 minutes or until crisp and browned; let cool.

2. Meanwhile, dice tomato, cucumber and bell pepper. Thinly slice onion. Reserve ¼ cup of the tomato, 2 tablespoons each of the cucumber and bell pepper, and 1 tablespoon of the onion for dressing. Place torn leaf lettuce in medium bowl.

3. In blender combine reserved tomato, cucumber, bell pepper, onion, olive oil, vinegar, garlic, salt and cayenne. Puree until well blended; strain. Reserve ¼ cup of the dressing. Toss lettuce with remaining dressing; divide evenly among 6 salad plates. Sprinkle remaining tomato, cucumber, bell pepper and onion evenly over lettuce; drizzle with reserved dressing. Top with croutons.

6 servings.
Preparation time: 25 minutes. Ready to serve: 25 minutes.

Per serving: 185 calories, 14 g total fat (2.5 g saturated fat), 15 mg cholesterol, 270 mg sodium, 2.5 g fiber.

WINTER SALAD WITH ENDIVE AND CELERY ROOT

Belgian endive and celery root are both popular ingredients in Parisian salads. To prepare ahead, make vinaigrette and assemble lettuce, endive and celery root. To keep the celery root from darkening, toss with enough vinaigrette to coat. Refrigerate vinaigrette, lettuce, endive and celery root. Toss to combine just before serving.

VINAIGRETTE
- 2 tablespoons Dijon mustard
- 3 tablespoons white wine vinegar
- 2/3 cup vegetable oil
- 1/4 teaspoon salt
- 1/8 teaspoon freshly ground pepper

SALAD
- 4 cups mixed leaf lettuce
- 1 head Belgian endive, cut into 1/2-inch slices
- 1 cup diced celery root

1 In small bowl, whisk together mustard and vinegar. Slowly whisk in oil; season with salt and pepper.

2 In large bowl, combine lettuce, endive and celery root. Toss with vinaigrette to coat.

4 to 6 servings.
Preparation time: 20 minutes. Ready to serve: 20 minutes.

Per 4 servings: 360 calories, 37 g total fat (5.5 g saturated fat), 0 mg cholesterol, 280 mg sodium, 5 g fiber.

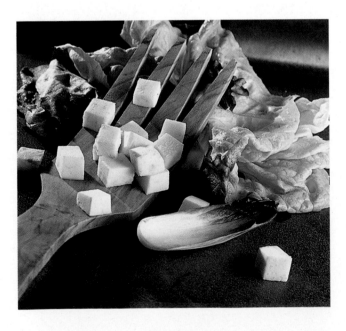

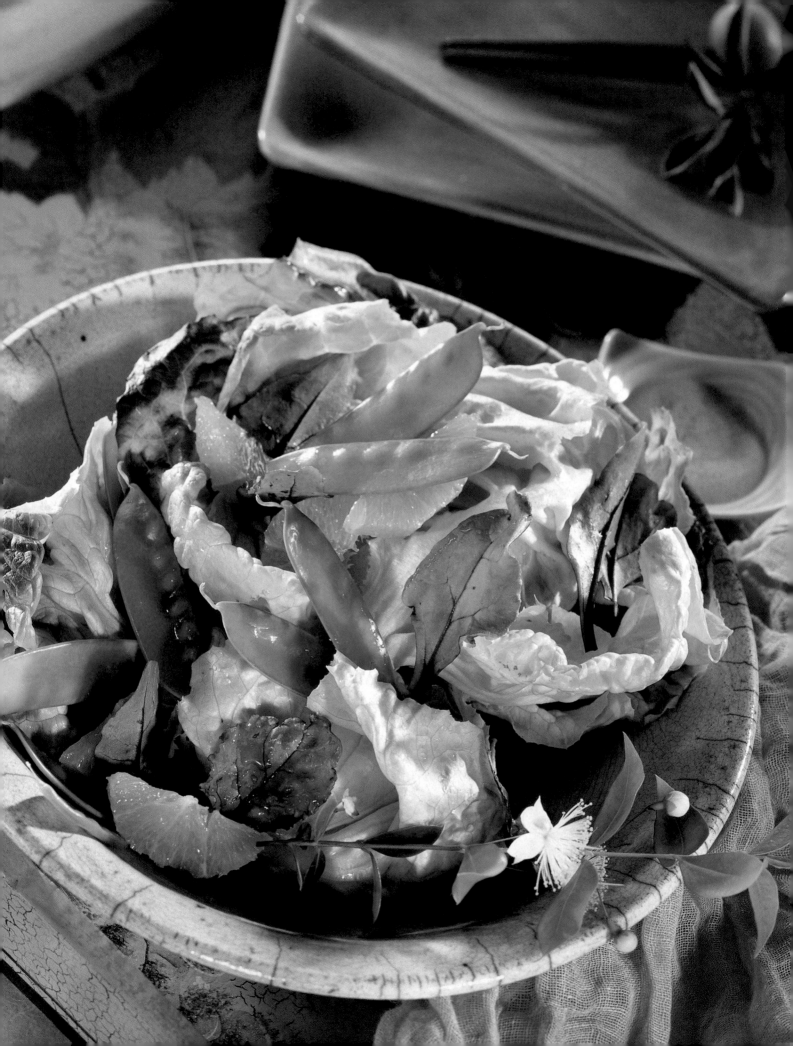

SPICY PEA POD AND ORANGE SALAD

In the early spring, substitute several handfuls of pea shoots from the market for the pea pods. Tahini is a ground sesame paste. If you have trouble finding it, use peanut butter instead.

VINAIGRETTE
- 2 tablespoons cider vinegar
- 1 tablespoon tahini
- 1 teaspoon honey
- 1/2 teaspoon hot pepper sauce
- 1/4 teaspoon salt
- 1/3 cup vegetable oil

SALAD
- 1/2 lb. pea pods
- 6 cups mixed organic greens
- 2 oranges or tangerines, peeled, divided into segments

❶ In small bowl, whisk together vinegar, tahini, honey, hot pepper sauce and salt. Slowly whisk in oil.

❷ Bring a large saucepan half-filled with water to a boil over high heat. Add pea pods; cook 30 to 60 seconds or until pea pods turn a vivid green. Drain; run under cold water to stop cooking; pat dry. Place greens in large bowl; toss with dressing. Top with pea pods and orange segments. Serve immediately.

6 servings.
Preparation time: 10 minutes. Ready to serve: 10 minutes.

Per serving: 165 calories, 13.5 g total fat (2 g saturated fat), 0 mg cholesterol, 105 mg sodium, 3 g fiber.

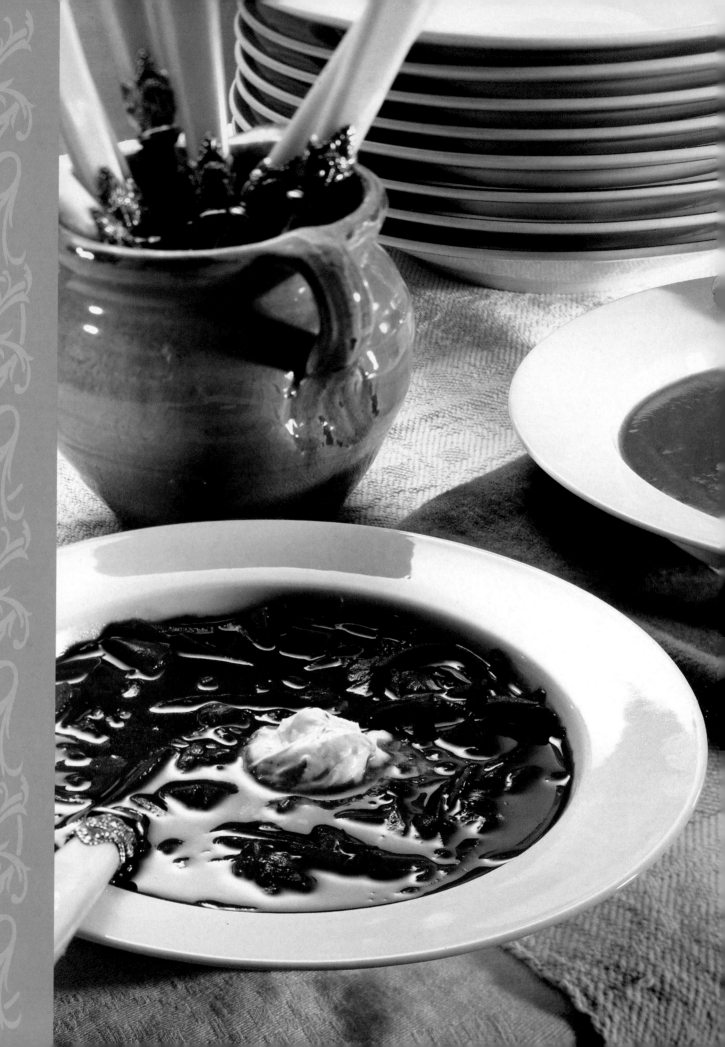

SOUPS

The soup pot is an ideal destination for vegetables. Their inherent moisture and intense flavors make them natural additions. Start with some broth or stock and see what the refrigerator has to offer. Throw in some pasta, canned beans or cream to make the finished product even more satisfying. Before you know it, people will be asking you for the recipe.

Borscht with Double Caraway Cream, page 58
Carrot, Orange and Ginger Soup, page 59

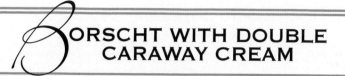

BORSCHT WITH DOUBLE CARAWAY CREAM

Charnuska is a small, black seed used in Indian cooking. Also known as black caraway, it is used to top Jewish rye.

CREAM
- 1/2 cup sour cream
- 1/2 teaspoon caraway seeds, lightly crushed
- 1/4 teaspoon charnuska, if desired

BORSCHT
- 2 tablespoons vegetable oil
- 1 large onion, chopped
- 1 teaspoon minced garlic
- 1/2 medium cabbage, shredded
- 2 medium beets, shredded
- 6 cups beef broth or *Rich Vegetable Stock* (page 61)
- 1 (14.5-oz.) can diced tomatoes, undrained
- 3 tablespoons red wine vinegar
- 1/2 teaspoon freshly ground pepper
- 1/2 teaspoon celery salt
- 1 medium potato, cut into 1/2-inch pieces

❶ In small bowl, combine sour cream, caraway and charnuska. Let sit overnight for all flavors to blend.*

❷ Heat oil in nonreactive Dutch oven over medium heat until hot. Add onion; sauté 4 to 5 minutes or until softened. Add garlic; sauté an additional minute or until fragrant. Add cabbage, beets, broth, tomatoes, vinegar, pepper and celery salt. Bring to a boil; reduce heat to low. Simmer, covered, 1 1/2 hours. Add potato during last 45 minutes of cooking. Serve with Double Caraway Cream.

TIP *If unable to do in advance, combine caraway seeds with 2 teaspoons of very hot water; let sit while preparing remainder of recipe. Combine with sour cream and charnuska before serving.

6 main course or 8 first course servings.
Preparation time: 25 minutes. Ready to serve: 8 hours, 25 minutes.

Per main course serving: 180 calories, 9 g total fat (3 g saturated fat), 15 mg cholesterol, 1315 mg sodium, 4 g fiber.

CARROT, ORANGE AND GINGER SOUP

Perfect on a hot summer day, this cold soup bursts with flavor. The acidity of the orange plays against the sweetness of the carrots and the spicy sharpness of the ginger.

5	cups *Light Vegetable Stock* (page 60) or 5 cups water
1	lb. carrots, peeled, cut into 1-inch pieces
2	teaspoons grated fresh ginger
1/4	cup thawed orange juice concentrate
1	teaspoon salt
1/8	teaspoon freshly ground pepper

❶ In Dutch oven, bring stock, carrots and ginger to a boil over medium-high heat. Reduce heat to low; simmer, partially covered, 40 to 45 minutes or until carrots are very tender. Remove from heat; cool slightly. Puree carrots and cooking liquid in blender or food processor. Stir in orange juice concentrate, salt and pepper. Chill 3 to 4 hours or overnight.

4 servings.
Preparation time: 15 minutes. Ready to serve: 4 hours.

Per serving: 90 calories, .5 g total fat (0 g saturated fat), 0 mg cholesterol, 620 mg sodium, 3.5 g fiber.

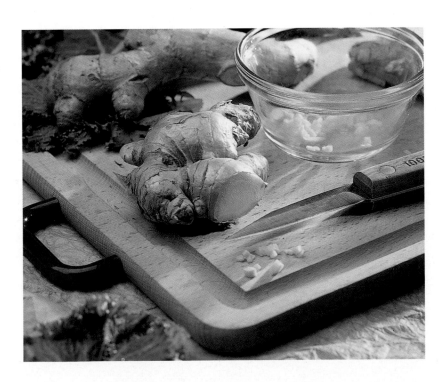

LIGHT VEGETABLE STOCK

This light stock adds flavor to soups and dishes where chicken broth would normally be used. When substituting for canned broth, add 1/4 to 1/2 teaspoon of salt for every cup used.

1	large onion, peeled, halved
2	large carrots, cut into large pieces
1	rib celery, cut into large pieces
1	medium potato, halved
1	bunch green onions
6	stems parsley
1	bay leaf
2	sprigs fresh thyme or 1/2 teaspoon dried
3 to 4	peppercorns
9	cups water

❶ Place all ingredients in Dutch oven. Bring to a boil over medium-high heat. Reduce heat to low; barely simmer, partially covered, 2 hours. Strain. Refrigerate up to 3 days or freeze.

6 cups.
Preparation time: 10 minutes. Ready to serve: 2 hours, 10 minutes.
Per cup: 10 calories, 0 g total fat (0 g saturated fat), 0 mg cholesterol, 5 mg sodium, 0 g fiber.

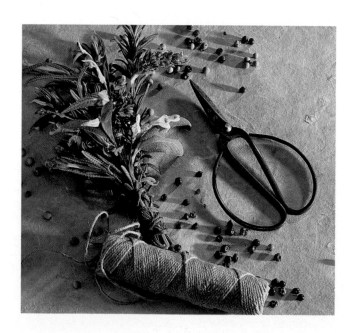

RICH VEGETABLE STOCK

This homemade stock adds richness and color. Use it as a substitute for beef stocks and broths in recipes. As with the light vegetable stock, if substituting for canned broth, add 1/4 to 1/2 teaspoon of salt for every cup used.

1 large onion, cut in quarters, outer skin removed
1 medium tomato, halved
1 rib celery, cut into large pieces
1 large carrot, cut into large pieces
1 medium potato, halved
1 bunch green onions
1 tablespoon vegetable oil
9 cups water
6 parsley stems
2 sprigs fresh thyme or 1/2 teaspoon dried
3 to 4 peppercorns
1 bay leaf
2 tablespoons soy sauce

❶ Heat oven to 400°F. Place onion, tomato, celery, carrot, potato and green onions in large shallow roasting or baking pan. Drizzle with oil; toss to coat. Bake 30 to 40 minutes or until browned, turning every 10 minutes to prevent burning. Remove vegetables; place in large pot.

❷ Add 1 cup water to roasting pan. Cook on low heat, scraping up any brown bits from bottom of pan. Pour mixture into large pot.

❸ To vegetable mixture, add parsley, thyme, peppercorns, bay leaf, remaining 8 cups water and soy sauce. Bring to a boil over medium-high heat. Reduce heat to low; simmer, partially covered, 2 hours. Strain; refrigerate up to 3 days or freeze.

6 cups.
Preparation time: 10 minutes. Ready to serve: 2 hours, 40 minutes.
Per cup: 40 calories, 2.5 g total fat (.5 g saturated fat), 0 mg cholesterol, 350 mg sodium, .5 g fiber.

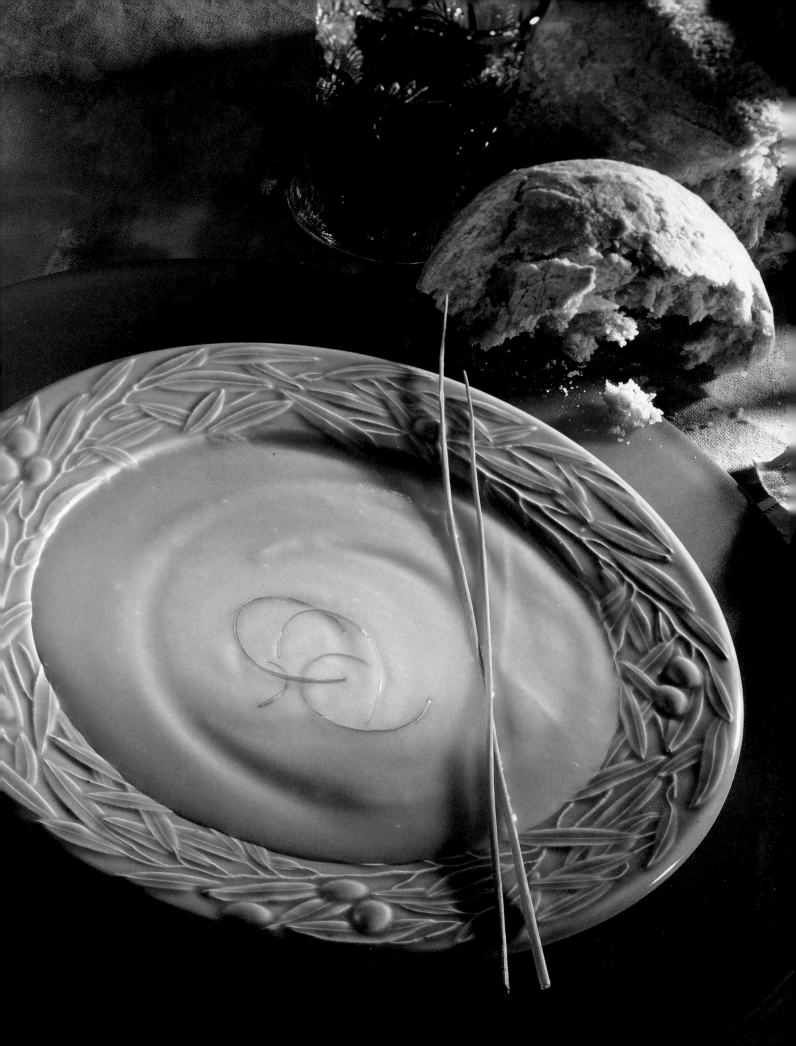

CREAMY THREE-POTATO SOUP

Soups can be creamy without a lot of added fat. The pureed potatoes give this soup a rich, velvety texture accented by the subtle flavor of leeks. To clean leeks, trim off root ends and cut the stalks in half lengthwise. Separate sections under running water to remove grit.

2 tablespoons vegetable oil
2 medium leeks, chopped, white and light green portions only
1 medium onion, sliced
6 cups reduced-sodium chicken broth (or 6 cups
   Light Vegetable Stock (page 60) plus 1¼ teaspoons salt)
½ lb. russet potatoes, peeled, sliced
½ lb. Yukon Gold potatoes, peeled, sliced
1 lb. sweet potatoes or yams, peeled, sliced
½ cup milk
¼ teaspoon white pepper

❶ Heat oil in Dutch oven over medium heat until hot. Sauté leeks and onion 3 to 4 minutes. Add broth and potatoes; bring to a boil. Reduce heat to low; simmer, partially covered, about 30 to 40 minutes, or until tender. Remove from heat; cool slightly. Puree in blender or food processor; return to Dutch oven. Stir in milk and pepper. Heat gently over low heat just until hot.

6 main course or 8 first course servings.
Preparation time: 25 minutes. Ready to serve: 1 hour.

Per main course serving: 225 calories, 6.5 g total fat (1.5 g saturated fat), 0 mg cholesterol, 505 mg sodium, 4 g fiber.

CHEDDAR AND VEGETABLE SOUP

This variation on beer cheese soup is hearty and comforting. Make sure to include some of the broccoli stems as well as the buds. Peel the stems before using if the outer skin is tough.

1/4 cup butter
1 medium onion, chopped (about 1 cup)
1 rib celery, chopped (about 1/2 cup)
1/2 cup all-purpose flour
1 (14.5-oz) can reduced-sodium chicken broth
     (or 2 cups *Light Vegetable Stock* (page 60) plus 1/2 teaspoon salt)
2 cups milk
1 medium potato, diced
3 cups chopped broccoli
1 cup beer
8 oz. grated extra-sharp cheddar cheese (about 2 cups)
1 teaspoon Worcestershire sauce
1/2 teaspoon salt
1/8 teaspoon hot pepper sauce

❶ Melt butter in Dutch oven over medium heat. Add onion and celery; sauté 4 to 5 minutes or until softened. Stir in flour. Whisk in broth and milk. Add potato; slowly bring to a boil, stirring occasionally. Reduce heat to low; simmer, partially covered, 10 minutes, stirring occasionally. Stir in broccoli and beer; continue cooking partially covered an additional 15 minutes, stirring occasionally. Stir in cheese, Worcestershire sauce, salt and hot pepper sauce. Serve hot.

6 servings.
Preparation time: 20 minutes. Ready to serve: 45 minutes.
Per serving: 360 calories, 22.5 g total fat (14 g saturated fat), 65 mg cholesterol, 695 mg sodium, 2.5 g fiber.

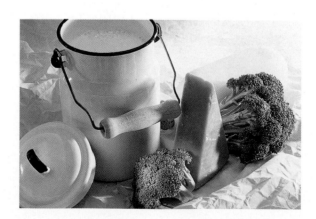

HERBED LENTIL SOUP

Serve this soup on a cold winter day. Use canned tomatoes for ease of preparation. If you want to use fresh tomatoes, all the better; the tip at the end of this recipe tells you what to substitute.

2   tablespoons olive oil
2   medium onions, chopped (about 2 cups)
2   large carrots, chopped (about 1 cup)
3/4   teaspoon dried thyme
1/2   teaspoon dried oregano
4   cups reduced-sodium chicken broth (or 4 cups
      Light Vegetable Stock (page 60) plus 1 teaspoon salt)
1/2   cup dry red wine
1   cup lentils, rinsed
1   (14.5-oz.) can diced tomatoes, undrained*
2   tablespoons chopped fresh parsley

❶ Heat oil in nonreactive Dutch oven over medium heat until hot. Add onions and carrots; sauté 4 to 5 minutes. Add thyme and oregano; sauté an additional minute. Add broth, wine, lentils and tomatoes. Bring to a boil; reduce heat to low. Simmer, partially covered, 40 to 45 minutes or until lentils are tender. Garnish with fresh chopped parsley.

TIP *One pound chopped, peeled tomatoes plus 1/2 teaspoon salt may be substituted for the canned tomatoes.

6 main course servings.
Preparation time: 15 minutes. Ready to serve: 55 minutes.
Per serving: 220 calories, 6 g total fat (1 g saturated fat), 0 mg cholesterol, 450 mg sodium, 10 g fiber.

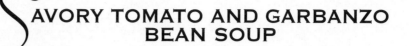

SAVORY TOMATO AND GARBANZO BEAN SOUP

A fabulous soup served poolside at the Steltzner Vineyards in the Napa Valley inspired this recipe.

- 2 tablespoons olive oil
- 1 large onion, chopped
- 6 large basil leaves
- 4 large sage leaves
- 4 sprigs Italian parsley
  Leaves from 2-inch sprig rosemary
- 2 large garlic cloves, minced
- 1 (15-oz.) can garbanzo beans, drained, rinsed
- 5 medium tomatoes, chopped, juice reserved
- 1 (14.5-oz.) can reduced-sodium chicken broth (or 2 cups
  Light Vegetable Stock (page 60) plus 1/2 teaspoon salt)
- 1/8 teaspoon freshly ground pepper

❶ Heat oil in nonreactive Dutch oven over medium heat until hot. Add onion; sauté about 5 minutes, stirring often.

❷ Meanwhile, chop basil, sage, parsley and rosemary together. When onion is softened, add herbs, garlic and beans. Sauté an additional 2 to 3 minutes. Remove half of bean mixture from Dutch oven; reserve.

❸ To Dutch oven, add tomatoes and their juice, broth and pepper; bring to a boil. Reduce heat to medium-low; cook an additional 15 minutes. Remove from heat; puree in blender or food processor. Return to Dutch oven; stir in reserved bean mixture. Bring to a simmer over medium heat.

4 main course or 6 first course servings.
Preparation time: 30 minutes. Ready to serve: 50 minutes.

Per main course serving: 245 calories, 10 g total fat (1.5 g saturated fat), 0 mg cholesterol, 410 mg sodium, 6.5 g fiber.

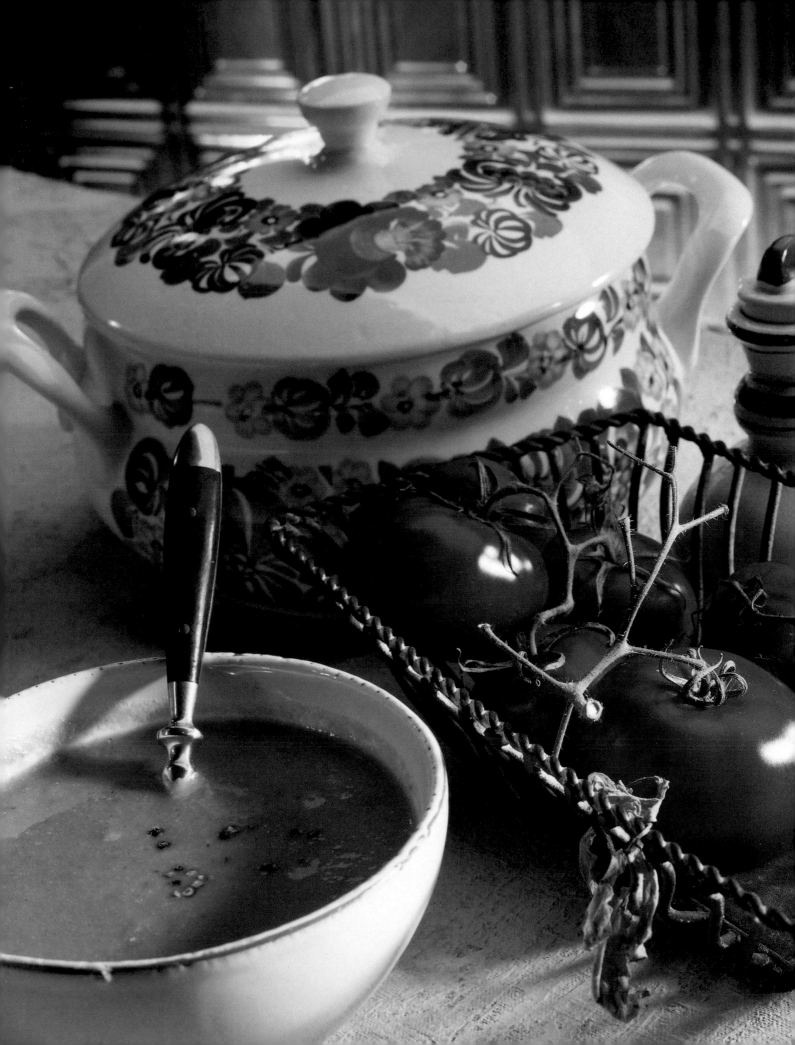

SPRING ASPARAGUS SOUP

If you are a frugal cook, save the woody ends trimmed from asparagus in other recipes and use them as part of the asparagus called for here. Crème fraîche is a thick, rich, nutty cream available in gourmet supermarkets. Substitute sour cream if unavailable, but do not allow it to boil.

1	tablespoon butter
1/4	cup chopped shallots
2	lb. asparagus
4	cups reduced-sodium chicken broth (or 4 cups *Light Vegetable Stock* (page 60) plus 1 teaspoon salt)
1/4	cup plus 2 tablespoons crème fraîche
6	spinach leaves, cut into ribbons

❶ In Dutch oven, melt butter over medium heat. Add shallots; sauté 3 to 4 minutes or until softened. Remove tips from asparagus; reserve. Cut spears into 2-inch pieces; add to Dutch oven. Add broth; bring to a boil. Reduce heat to low; simmer 10 minutes or until spears are tender.

❷ Remove asparagus mixture from heat; puree in blender. Strain; return to Dutch oven. Add 1/4 cup of the crème fraîche and asparagus tips; simmer 3 to 5 minutes or until asparagus is crisp-tender. If using sour cream, heat through but do not boil. Ladle into bowls; top each bowl with 1 teaspoon of the crème fraîche and 1 spinach leaf.

6 servings.
Preparation time: 20 minutes. Ready to serve: 35 minutes.

Per serving: 110 calories, 8 g total fat (4.5 g saturated fat), 20 mg cholesterol, 350 mg sodium, 1.5 g fiber.

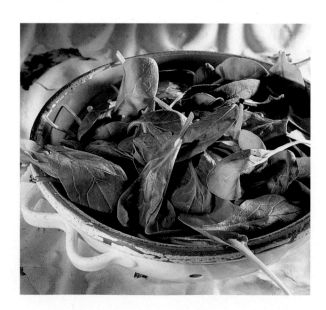

ONION SOUP

Don't be tempted to hurry the onions. They give the soup its distinctive flavor.

3	tablespoons vegetable oil
4	large onions, thinly sliced (about 8 cups)
1 1/2	teaspoons sugar
1/4	teaspoon salt
1/8	teaspoon pepper
5	cups beef broth plus 1 cup water (or 3 cups *Rich Vegetable Stock* (page 61) plus 1 teaspoon salt)
1/2	cup dry white wine
6 to 8	slices stale baguette (1 inch thick), toasted
1 1/2	cups (6 oz.) shredded Gruyère or Emmentaler cheese

❶ Heat oil in nonreactive Dutch oven over medium-high heat until hot. Add onions; stir to coat. Sauté 5 to 7 minutes until onions begin to soften, turning occasionally. Reduce heat to low; sprinkle with sugar; cover and cook 30 minutes, stirring occasionally. Uncover; increase heat to medium. Continue cooking 20 to 25 minutes or until onions turn a rich brown. (As onions begin to brown, scrape bottom of pan with a wooden spoon to incorporate caramel color into onions and to prevent scorching.) Stir in broth and wine; bring to a boil. Reduce heat to low; simmer, partially covered, 30 minutes. Season with salt and pepper, if desired.

❷ Heat broiler; ladle hot soup into oven-proof bowls. Top with 1 slice bread for first course serving or 2 for main course; sprinkle with cheese. Place bowls on baking sheet; broil until cheese is melted.

4 main course or 6 first course servings.
Preparation time: 40 minutes. Ready to serve: 1 hour, 45 minutes.

Per main course serving: 415 calories, 23 g total fat (9.5 g saturated fat), 40 mg cholesterol, 1690 mg sodium, 3.5 g fiber.

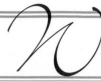

WILD RICE AND MUSHROOM SOUP

Wild rice is not really a rice but rather a marsh grass. It adds a wonderful, nutty flavor to this soup. Pancetta is a cured, unsmoked Italian bacon. If unavailable, substitute regular bacon, simmering it in water for 10 minutes to remove the smoky flavor. Drain and thoroughly pat dry before using. Vegetarians can omit the pancetta and increase the oil to three tablespoons.

1 (1-oz.) pkg. dried wild mushrooms
1 cup very hot water (115°F to 120°F)
1 tablespoon vegetable oil
1 cup diced pancetta
1/4 cup chopped shallots or green onions
1 (8-oz.) pkg. mushrooms, sliced
1/3 cup all-purpose flour
2 cups milk
1 (14.5-oz.) can chicken broth (or an additional 2 cups milk
    plus 3/4 teaspoon salt)
2 cups cooked wild rice*

❶ Soak dried mushrooms in very hot water in medium bowl 30 minutes. Remove mushrooms; chop. Strain soaking liquid through coffee filter to remove grit; set aside.

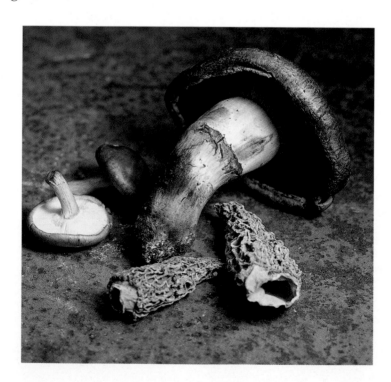

② Heat oil in Dutch oven over medium-high heat until hot. Add pancetta; sauté 1 minute. Add shallots; sauté 3 to 5 minutes or until tender and pancetta is browned. Add mushrooms; sauté 5 to 8 minutes or until tender. Add chopped wild mushrooms and reserved soaking liquid. Cook 5 minutes or until all liquid is absorbed. Stir in flour; whisk in milk and broth. Bring to a boil; continue cooking, stirring, for several minutes to thicken. Stir in rice; reduce heat to low. Simmer 5 minutes.

TIP *To cook wild rice, rinse 3/4 cup wild rice under cold water. Place in medium saucepan with 2 1/2 cups water. Add 3/4 teaspoon salt. Bring to a boil over medium-high heat. Reduce heat to low; cover and cook 45 to 60 minutes or until grains have opened and rice is chewy-tender. Drain if necessary.

4 main course or 6 first course servings.
Preparation time: 30 minutes. Ready to serve: 1 hour, 20 minutes.
Per main course serving: 295 calories, 11 g total fat (3.5 g saturated fat), 15 mg cholesterol, 905 mg sodium, 3 g fiber.

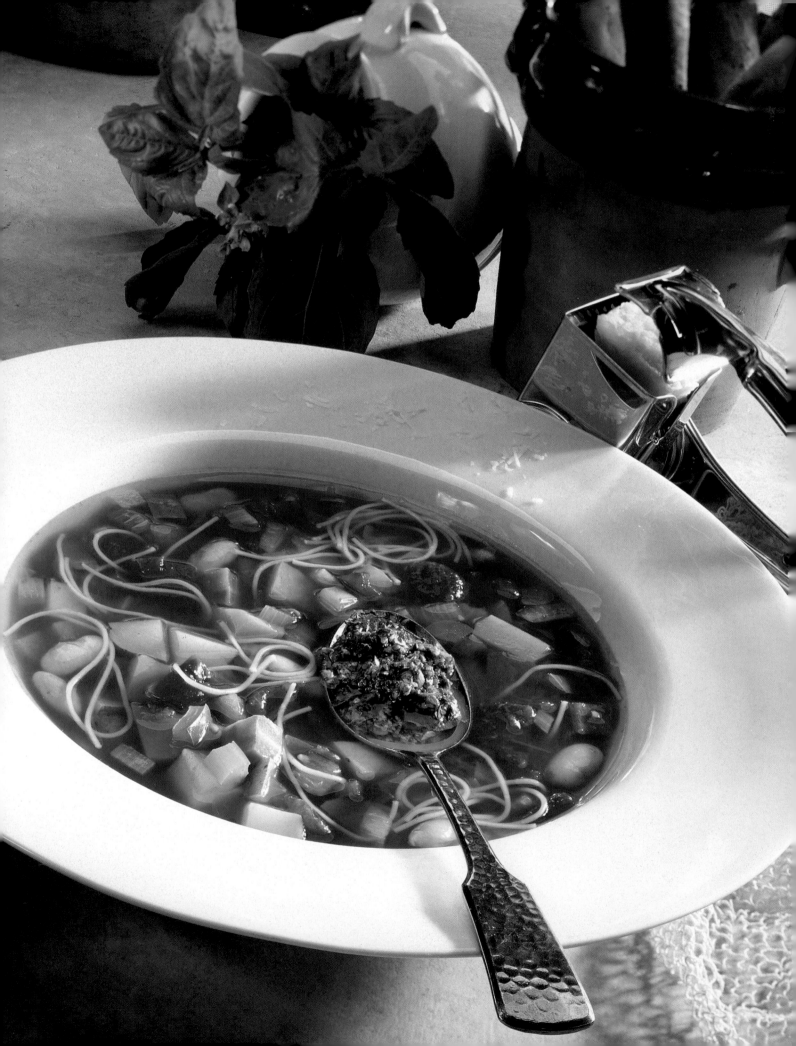

WINTER SOUP AU PISTOU

Pistou is the French equivalent of pesto. Make pistou (or pesto) in the summertime when fresh basil is abundant; freeze in small amounts to savor during the colder months.

2 tablespoons extra-virgin olive oil
1 medium onion, chopped
1½ teaspoons minced garlic
1 cup cubed peeled butternut squash
1 green bell pepper, diced
1 rib celery, chopped
1 medium carrot, chopped
1 small potato, cubed
6 cups *Light Vegetable Stock* (page 60)
1 (14.5-oz.) can diced tomatoes, undrained
1 (15-oz.) can cannellini beans, drained, rinsed
½ cup broken vermicelli or capellini
¾ teaspoon salt
¼ teaspoon freshly ground pepper

PISTOU
1 cup packed fresh basil
½ cup fresh parsley, leaves only
1 teaspoon chopped garlic
¼ cup (1 oz.) freshly grated Parmesan cheese
¼ cup extra-virgin olive oil

❶ Heat 2 tablespoons oil in nonreactive Dutch oven over medium heat until hot. Add onion; sauté 4 to 5 minutes or until softened. Add 1½ teaspoons garlic; sauté 1 minute or until fragrant. Add squash, bell pepper, celery, carrot and potato; stir to combine. Add stock and tomatoes; stir to combine. Bring to a boil; reduce heat to low. Simmer, partially covered, 20 minutes. Add beans, vermicelli, salt and pepper. Simmer an additional 5 minutes.

❷ In food processor, combine basil, parsley and 1 teaspoon garlic; pulse to combine. Add cheese; pulse several times. With motor running, slowly pour in ¼ cup olive oil. To serve, spoon 1 tablespoon pistou into center of each bowl of soup. Pass extra in small bowl.

8 servings.
Preparation time: 45 minutes. Ready to serve: 1 hour, 10 minutes.
Per serving: 230 calories, 12 g total fat (2 g saturated fat), 5 mg cholesterol, 655 mg sodium, 5.5 g fiber.

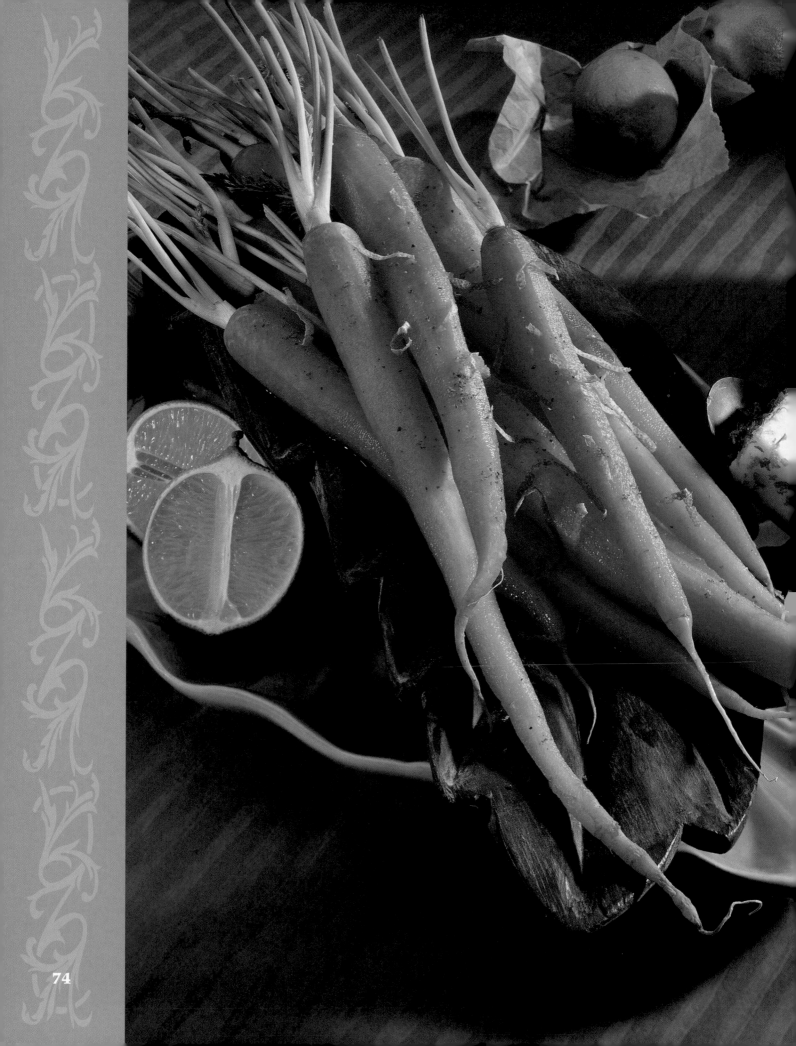

SIDES

Sometimes the sidekick should be the star. In terms of interest, the supporting role is sometimes the strongest. So it is with vegetable side dishes. Often downplayed, they can instead become the highlight of a meal. A simple main dish becomes a winner when paired with a flavorful side. Use these recipes and the tips in the Technique & Tools section to serve up the following scene (or plate) stealers.

Caribbean Carrots with Lime Butter, page 76

CARIBBEAN CARROTS WITH LIME BUTTER

Allspice, sometimes referred to as Jamaican pepper, is the berry of the evergreen tree. Along with the lime and hot sauce, the allspice gives a characteristic Caribbean flavor.

1/4 cup water
2 tablespoons sugar
2 teaspoons grated lime peel
1/2 teaspoon ground allspice
1/4 teaspoon ground nutmeg
1/4 teaspoon salt
1/8 teaspoon hot pepper sauce
1 (1-lb.) pkg. baby carrots or 2 lbs. fresh carrots, trimmed
2 tablespoons butter

❶ In medium saucepan, bring water, sugar, 1 teaspoon of the lime peel, allspice, nutmeg, salt and hot pepper sauce to a boil over medium heat. Add carrots; stir to coat. Reduce heat to low; cover and cook 8 to 10 minutes or until carrots are almost tender.

❷ Uncover; increase heat to high. Cook until cooking liquid evaporates, stirring often. Remove from heat; toss with butter and remaining 1 teaspoon lime peel.

6 servings.
Preparation time: 10 minutes. Ready to serve: 18 minutes.

Per serving: 85 calories, 4 g total fat (2.5 g saturated fat), 10 mg cholesterol, 150 mg sodium, 2.5 g fiber.

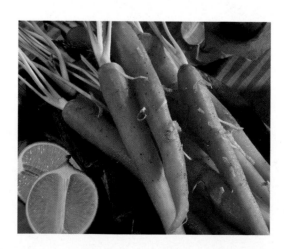

CONFETTI RISOTTO

Serve this colorful risotto as a side dish or on its own as a main course.

5	cups water
1	large carrot, cut into 1/2-inch pieces (about 1/2 cup)
1/2	red bell pepper, cut into 1/2-inch pieces (about 1/2 cup)
1/2	medium yellow squash, cut into 1/2-inch pieces (about 1/2 cup)
1/2	cup shelled peas
1/2	cup white wine
1	tablespoon soy sauce
1/8	teaspoon salt
2	tablespoons butter
1	small onion, chopped
1 1/2	cups arborio rice
1/2	cup (2 oz.) freshly grated Parmesan cheese

❶ Bring water to a boil in medium saucepan over medium-high heat. Add carrot; cook 5 minutes. Add bell pepper, squash and peas; cook an additional 5 minutes. Drain vegetables, reserving water. Set aside vegetables; return water to saucepan. Add wine, soy sauce and salt. Reduce heat to low; cover and keep wine mixture simmering while making risotto.

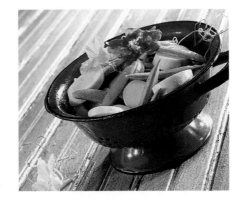

❷ Melt butter in large heavy saucepan over medium heat. Add onion; cook 4 to 5 minutes or until tender. Stir in rice; cook 2 to 3 minutes. Reduce heat to medium-low; add 1 cup wine mixture. Cook until liquid is absorbed, stirring often. Continue to add wine mixture 1 cup at a time, cooking and stirring often until rice is just slightly resistant to the bite and creamy, about 30 minutes. Stir in reserved vegetables and cheese.

6 side dish or 4 main dish servings.
Preparation time: 50 minutes. Ready to serve: 1 hour.

Per side dish serving: 280 calories, 7 g total fat (4.5 g saturated fat), 20 mg cholesterol, 440 mg sodium, 2.5 g fiber.

CORN RELISH

Bring this tasty relish to your next summer potluck. It's great with brats and hamburgers. For more elegant fare, try it with grilled salmon.

- 1/2 cup water
- 1/2 cup cider vinegar
- 1/3 cup sugar
- 3 cups corn (about 6 medium ears)
- 1 red bell pepper, chopped
- 1 small onion, halved, thinly sliced
- 1 Anaheim or New Mexico chile, seeded, chopped
- 2 teaspoons salt
- 1 teaspoon mustard seeds
- 1/2 teaspoon celery seeds
- 1/2 teaspoon ground turmeric
- 1/4 teaspoon hot pepper sauce
- 4 teaspoons all-purpose flour

❶ Bring all ingredients except 1/4 cup of the water and flour to a boil in large saucepan over medium-high heat. Reduce heat to low; simmer 5 minutes. In small bowl, whisk flour into remaining 1/4 cup water; stir into relish. Cook an additional 2 minutes to thicken. Spoon into clean jars. Store in refrigerator up to 2 weeks.

4 cups.
Preparation time: 15 minutes. Ready to serve: 22 minutes.
Per cup: 200 calories, 1 g total fat (0 g saturated fat), 0 mg cholesterol, 1175 mg sodium, 4 g fiber.

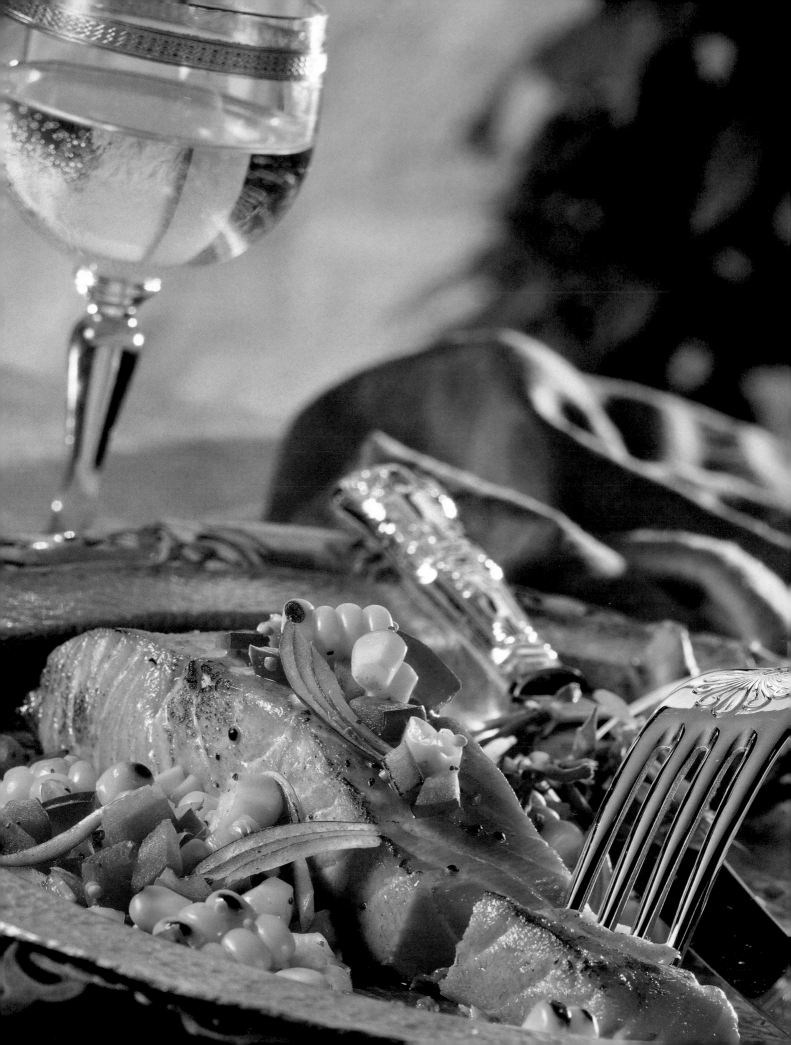

RAISED BEANS IN HOISIN SAUCE

Hoisin sauce is a flavorful ingredient common to Asian cooking. Look for it in your supermarket or in Asian grocery stores.

1 tablespoon vegetable oil
2 teaspoons minced garlic
2 teaspoons minced fresh ginger
1 lb. green beans, trimmed
1/2 cup water
1/4 cup hoisin sauce

❶ Heat oil in large nonstick skillet over medium-high heat until hot. Add garlic and ginger; sauté 30 to 60 seconds or until fragrant. Immediately add green beans; toss to coat.

❷ Combine water and hoisin sauce in small bowl. Pour over beans. Reduce heat to low; cover and cook 20 to 25 minutes, or until beans are tender and sauce has thickened enough to coat beans, stirring occasionally. If beans finish cooking before sauce has thickened, remove them from the skillet; place on large bowl. Increase heat to high; reduce sauce slightly to thicken. Pour sauce over beans.

4 servings.
Preparation time: 15 minutes. Ready to serve: 35 minutes.

Per serving: 90 calories, 4.5 g total fat (.5 g saturated fat), 0 mg cholesterol, 10 mg sodium, 3.5 g fiber.

GARLIC SCALLOPED POTATOES WITH PARMESAN CRUMB CRUST

Cooking the freshly sliced potatoes with the milk thickens the mixture before baking it in the oven. Garlic gives the distinctive flavor and the crumbs add a nice crunch. Make your own bread crumbs by drying leftover bread. Pulse the bread in a food processor fitted with a metal blade to make fine crumbs.

1³/₄ cups milk
1 tablespoon chopped garlic
¹/₂ teaspoon salt
¹/₈ teaspoon freshly ground pepper
2 lb. Yukon Gold potatoes, peeled if desired, sliced
     ¹/₈ inch thick (about 6 cups)
¹/₃ cup dry bread crumbs
¹/₄ cup (1 oz.) freshly grated Parmesan cheese
1 tablespoon olive oil

❶ Heat oven to 375°F. Spray 8 x 12-inch (or 9 x 13-inch) baking dish with nonstick cooking spray. Heat milk, garlic, salt and pepper in Dutch oven over medium-low heat. Add potatoes; stir to coat. Bring to a simmer, stirring gently. Cook 2 to 3 minutes or until milk begins to thicken. Pour into baking dish. Bake 50 minutes or until potatoes are bubbling.

❷ In small bowl, combine bread crumbs and cheese. Add oil; toss to coat. Sprinkle bread crumb mixture over potatoes. Return to oven; cook an additional 15 to 20 minutes or until crumbs are browned and potatoes are tender.

6 servings.
Preparation time: 20 minutes. Ready to serve: 1 hour, 25 minutes.

Per serving: 235 calories, 5.5 g total fat (2 g saturated fat), 10 mg cholesterol, 380 mg sodium, 3 g fiber.

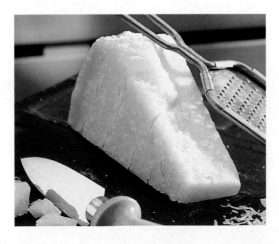

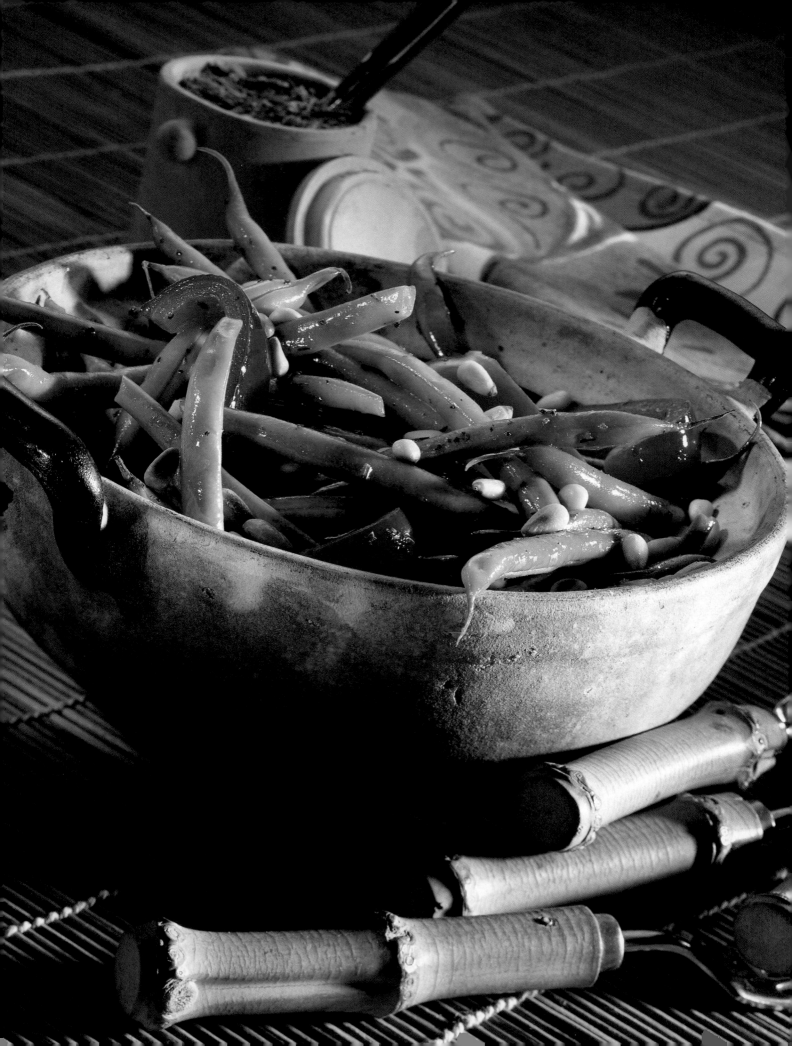

GREEN BEANS PROVENCALE

Herbes de Provence is a blend of dried spices common to the southern France area called Provence. The blend can vary in content, but usually contains thyme, savory, marjoram, basil and sometimes lavender. This dish can easily be doubled to serve a larger crowd; use a wok instead of a skillet to rewarm the beans.

- 2 lb. green beans, trimmed
- 2 tablespoons olive oil
- 1 red bell pepper, cut into strips
- 1 1/2 teaspoons herbes de Provence
- 1/4 teaspoon salt
- 1/4 cup pine nuts, toasted, if desired

1. Bring 2 quarts water to a boil in large pot over high heat. Add beans; return to a boil. Cook beans until crisp-tender, about 10 minutes. Drain; run under cold water to stop cooking. (Beans may be cooked ahead. Cover and refrigerate.)

2. Heat oil in large skillet over medium-high heat until hot. Add bell pepper; sauté 1 to 2 minutes. Add beans; cook 5 minutes or until heated, stirring occasionally. Sprinkle with herbes de Provence and salt; stir to coat. Serve topped with pine nuts.

8 servings.
Preparation time: 20 minutes. Ready to serve: 35 minutes.

Per serving: 80 calories, 6 g total fat (1 g saturated fat), 0 mg cholesterol, 85 mg sodium, 3.5 g fiber.

CHIPOTLE MASHED POTATOES

The buttery color of Yukon Gold potatoes make them seem extra rich. Serve with grilled chicken, fish or roast pork. For a vegetarian entrée, top with colorful stir-fried peppers and onions.

2 lb. Yukon Gold potatoes (3 to 4 medium), peeled, quartered
1 teaspoon salt
1 large garlic clove, peeled
1 chipotle pepper in adobo sauce, drained, finely minced
1/2 cup hot half-and-half or milk
2 tablespoons butter
1/2 teaspoon salt
1/8 teaspoon freshly ground pepper

❶ Place potatoes in large saucepan; add water to cover. Add salt and garlic; cook over medium heat 25 to 30 minutes or until potatoes are very tender. Drain; return potatoes and garlic to pan. Add pepper. Mash mixture until potatoes are fluffy and have no lumps. Stir in hot half-and-half and butter. Season with salt and pepper.

6 servings.
Preparation time: 15 minutes. Ready to serve: 40 minutes.
Per serving: 180 calories, 6.5 g total fat (4 g saturated fat), 20 mg cholesterol, 640 mg sodium, 2.5 g fiber.

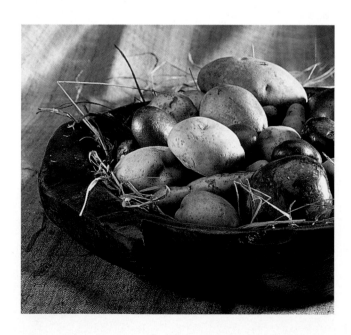

POTATO PANCAKES WITH ROSEMARY

Blanching the potatoes before frying gives them a perfect texture. Serve these pancakes with a dollop of sour cream or applesauce, if desired.

- 2 medium russet potatoes (about 3/4 lb.)
- 2 eggs, lightly beaten
- 1 tablespoon minced garlic
- 2 teaspoons minced fresh rosemary or 3/4 teaspoon dried
- 1/4 teaspoon salt
- 1/8 teaspoon freshly ground pepper
- 3 tablespoons oil

❶ Bring 2 quarts water to a boil in large pot over high heat. In food processor, shred potatoes to make 2 cups. Immediately drop potatoes into water; cook 1 minute. Strain; run under cold water to stop cooking. Place in towel; squeeze to remove excess moisture. Place in medium bowl; add eggs, garlic, rosemary, salt and pepper. Mix well.

❷ Heat 2 tablespoons of the oil in large skillet over medium-high heat until hot. Drop potato mixture by large mounded spoonfuls into skillet; flatten slightly to form 3-inch pancakes. Cook 7 to 9 minutes or until browned on both sides, turning once. Remove from skillet; set aside. Add remaining 1 tablespoon oil to pan; repeat with remaining potato mixture.

6 servings.
Preparation time: 13 minutes. Ready to serve: 27 minutes.

Per serving: 125 calories, 8.5 g total fat (1.5 g saturated fat), 70 mg cholesterol, 120 mg sodium, 1 g fiber.

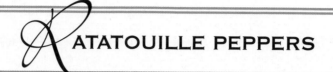

RATATOUILLE PEPPERS

Visit your local farmers' market in late summer to find the ingredients you need for this dish. Try serving these peppers with grilled tuna steaks. Turn them into a delicious vegetarian entrée by serving two stuffed pepper halves per person, along with a fresh, tossed salad and French bread.

- 3   tablespoons olive oil
- 1   large onion (about 1/2 lb.), chopped
- 1   tablespoon minced garlic
- 1/2   lb. peeled eggplant, cut into 1-inch pieces (3 cups)
- 1/2   lb. zucchini, cut into 1-inch pieces (2 cups)
- 1   yellow or orange bell pepper (about 1/2 lb.), cut into 1-inch pieces
- 2   large tomatoes (about 1 lb.), peeled, cut into 1-inch pieces
- 1/4   cup chopped fresh basil
- 1/2   teaspoon salt
- 1/4   teaspoon freshly ground pepper
- 3   red bell peppers, halved, seeded
- 3   tablespoons freshly grated Parmesan cheese

❶ Heat oil in nonreactive Dutch oven over medium-high heat until hot. Add onion; sauté 3 to 4 minutes or until softened. Add garlic; sauté an additional minute or until fragrant. Add eggplant, zucchini and yellow bell pepper; sauté an additional 4 to 5 minutes. Add tomatoes, basil, salt and pepper. Reduce heat to low; cook, covered, 15 minutes, stirring occasionally. Uncover; increase heat to medium. Cook about 10 to 15 minutes or until almost all cooking liquid has evaporated. Dish may be made up to 1 day ahead at this point. Cover and refrigerate.

❷ Heat oven to 350°F. Line baking sheet with foil. Place red bell peppers cut side up on baking sheet. Divide ratatouille mixture evenly among peppers. Top with cheese. Bake about 30 minutes or until peppers are crisp-tender and ratatouille is hot.

6 servings.
Preparation time: 40 minutes. Ready to serve: 1 hour, 25 minutes.

Per serving: 130 calories, 8 g total fat (1.5 g saturated fat), 0 mg cholesterol, 260 mg sodium, 3.5 g fiber.

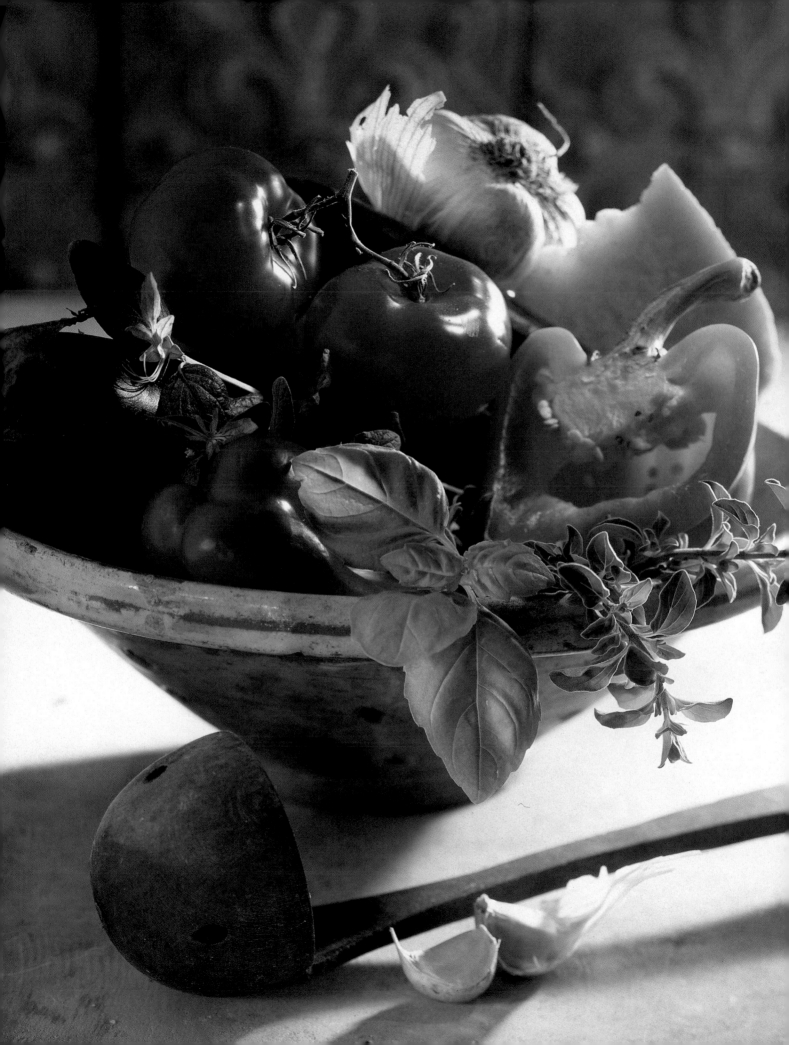

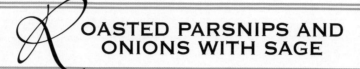

ROASTED PARSNIPS AND ONIONS WITH SAGE

Pair this side dish with roasted turkey or pork.

1 lb. parsnips (about 6 medium), peeled, cut in 1/4-inch slices
2 medium onions (about 3/4 lb.), sliced 1/2-inch thick
2 tablespoons olive oil
1 tablespoon honey
1 tablespoon balsamic vinegar
1 tablespoon finely chopped fresh sage
1/4 teaspoon salt
1/8 teaspoon freshly ground pepper

1 Heat oven to 400°F. Combine parsnips and onions in large bowl. In small bowl, stir together oil, honey and vinegar. Pour over vegetables; toss to coat. Spread vegetables on large shallow baking sheet. Bake 40 to 45 minutes, stirring every 15 minutes.

2 In small bowl, combine sage, salt and pepper. Toss vegetables with seasonings; return to oven. Cook an additional 2 to 3 minutes.

4 servings.
Preparation time: 10 minutes. Ready to serve: 52 minutes.

Per serving: 180 calories, 7 g total fat (1 g saturated fat), 0 mg cholesterol, 155 mg sodium, 5 g fiber.

SPICY MIXED GREENS

Check the glossary to see just how healthy this dish is for you. The crushed red pepper flakes and ginger accent the flavor of the mustard greens, and the tomato adds a bright color note.

2 tablespoons vegetable oil

1 large onion, chopped

1 tablespoon minced fresh ginger

1/2 teaspoon crushed red pepper flakes

1/2 cup reduced-sodium chicken broth or *Light Vegetable Stock* (page 60)

1 bunch collard greens (about 1 lb.), spines removed, cut into large pieces

1/2 bunch kale leaves (about 1/2 lb.), spines removed, cut into large pieces

1 bunch mustard greens (about 1/2 lb.), spines removed, cut into large pieces

1/4 teaspoon salt

1 large tomato, chopped

❶ Heat oil in nonreactive Dutch oven over medium-high heat until hot. Add onion; sauté 5 to 7 minutes or until onion softens and begins to brown. Add ginger and pepper flakes; sauté about 30 seconds. Add broth, collard greens and kale. Reduce heat to medium-low; cover and braise 10 minutes. (If Dutch oven is not large enough to accommodate all the greens at once, add as many as the pan will hold; cover for about one minute. As the greens in the pan shrink during cooking, add more greens until all the collard greens and kale have been added.)

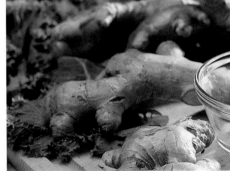

❷ Add mustard greens; braise, covered, an additional 10 minutes. Add salt and tomato; cook, uncovered, an additional 1 to 2 minutes or until tomato is just heated through. With slotted spoon, remove greens and tomato; place in large bowl.

❸ Increase heat to high; reduce remaining cooking juices until lightly syrupy. Toss with greens.

6 servings. Preparation time: 25 minutes. Ready to serve: 50 minutes.

Per serving: 95 calories, 5 g total fat (1 g saturated fat), 0 mg cholesterol, 165 mg sodium, 4 g fiber.

SESAME ASPARAGUS

Make sure you purchase toasted, dark sesame oil for use in this dish. Used as a flavoring agent in this or any other Asian cooking, it adds a rich, nutty flavor.

- 1 tablespoon oyster sauce
- 1 tablespoon soy sauce
- 1 tablespoon dry sherry or white wine
- 1 teaspoon cornstarch
- 1 1/2 teaspoons dark sesame oil
- 2 tablespoons sesame seeds
- 1 tablespoon vegetable oil
- 1 1/2 teaspoons minced fresh ginger
- 1 teaspoon minced garlic
- 1 lb. asparagus, trimmed, cut diagonally into 1 1/2-inch pieces
- 1 large carrot, cut diagonally into thin pieces
- 1/2 cup chicken broth or water
- 1 bunch green onions, cut diagonally into 1-inch pieces

❶ In small bowl, combine oyster sauce, soy sauce and sherry. Add cornstarch; stir to dissolve. Stir in sesame oil. Set aside.

❷ Place sesame seeds in unheated wok. Brown over medium heat until seeds turn golden, about 2 to 3 minutes. Remove seeds; set aside. Increase heat to high. Add oil; swirl to coat wok. Add ginger, garlic, asparagus and carrot. Stir-fry 2 minutes. Add broth; cover and cook an additional 2 minutes or until asparagus and carrot are almost crisp-tender. Uncover. Add green onions. Stir-fry an additional minute. Add oyster sauce mixture; stir until thickened. Toss with sesame seeds.

4 servings.
Preparation time: 30 minutes. Ready to serve: 30 minutes.

Per serving: 125 calories, 8 g total fat (1 g saturated fat), 0 mg cholesterol, 575 mg sodium, 3 g fiber.

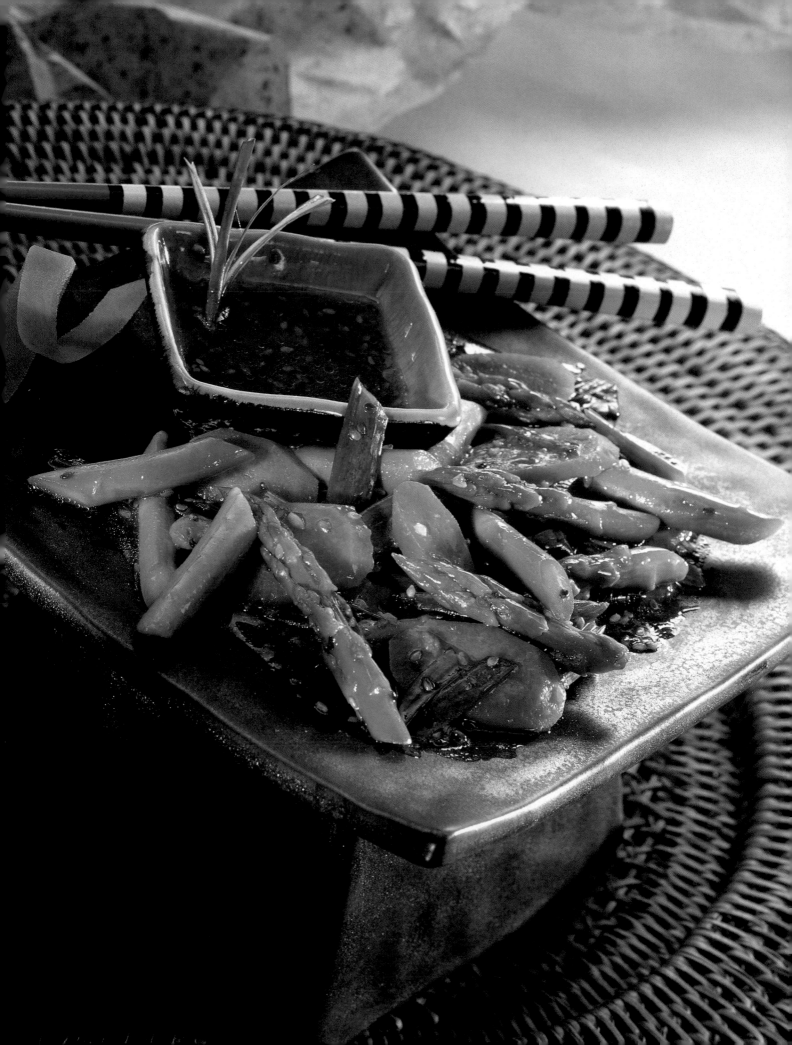

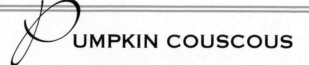

PUMPKIN COUSCOUS

Harissa* is a highly seasoned North African condiment available in specialty food shops. It adds extra heat and flavor to couscous and other regional dishes.

1	(10-oz.) pkg. couscous
2	cups *Light Vegetable Stock* (page 60) or water
3	medium tomatoes, chopped
1½	teaspoons ground ginger
½	teaspoon ground nutmeg
½	teaspoon ground allspice
½	teaspoon ground cardamom
½	teaspoon cinnamon
½	teaspoon turmeric
½	teaspoon salt
¼	teaspoon ground coriander
¼	teaspoon freshly ground black pepper
¼	teaspoon cayenne
1	(¾-pound) pumpkin, seeded, peeled, cut into 1½-inch chunks
10 to 12	baby carrots
1	medium onion, cut into 1½-inch chunks
1	turnip, cut into 1½-inch chunks
½	cup raisins

❶ Cook couscous according to package directions.

❷ In large saucepan, combine stock, tomatoes, ginger, nutmeg, allspice, cardamom, cinnamon, turmeric, salt, coriander, pepper and cayenne; mix well. Bring to a boil; add pumpkin, carrots, onion, turnip and just enough water to cover. Return to a boil. Reduce heat to simmer about 20 minutes or until vegetables are tender. Stir in raisins.

❸ On platter, make ring with couscous. Place vegetables in center; drizzle with broth. Serve remaining broth mixed with harissa, if desired.

TIP *Hot pepper sauce can be substituted.

4 to 6 servings.
Preparation time: 20 minutes. Ready to serve: 1 hour.

Per serving: 390 calories, 1.5 g total fat (.5 g saturated fat), 0 mg cholesterol, 330 mg sodium, 9 g fiber.

LEEK AND BOK CHOY GRATIN

Looking for a change from the ordinary? Simple to prepare,
this dish is amazingly good.

1   lb. leeks, white and pale green portions, cut into
       1¹/₂-inch pieces (about 4 cups)
1   lb. bok choy, stems and leaves, cut into 1¹/₂-inch pieces
       (about 5 cups)
¹/₂ cup chicken broth (or ¹/₂ cup water plus 1 tablespoon soy sauce)
1   tablespoon all-purpose flour
1   cup (4 oz.) grated Gruyère or other Swiss-style cheese

❶ Heat oven to 350°F. In large bowl, combine leeks and bok choy; toss.
Place in 8 x 12-inch (or 9 x 13-inch) baking dish.

❷ In small bowl, whisk together broth and flour. Pour over leek mixture.
Cover tightly with foil; bake 45 minutes, stirring once after 30 minutes.
Remove from oven. Stir; sprinkle with cheese. Return to oven,
uncovered; bake an additional 10 to 15 minutes or until cheese is
melted.

6 servings.
Preparation time: 10 minutes. Ready to serve: 1 hour, 5 minutes.

Per serving: 100 calories, 5.5 g total fat (3.5 g saturated fat), 15 mg cholesterol, 190 mg sodium, 1.5 g fiber.

SPINACH TIMBALES

Timbale refers to the round, high-sided mold that tapers slightly and is used for baking, as well as the dish that is baked in the mold. Timbale molds can be purchased in some specialty cookware stores. Custard cups provide an easier alternative. Using frozen spinach in this recipe speeds the cooking process without sacrificing taste.

TIMBALES
- 1 tablespoon butter
- 1/4 cup minced onion
- 1 1/2 teaspoons minced garlic
- 1 1/2 teaspoons minced fresh ginger
- 1/4 cup tomato sauce
- 1/2 tablespoon coriander
- 1/2 teaspoon cumin
- 1/4 teaspoon ground red pepper
- 1/4 teaspoon salt
- 1/8 teaspoon turmeric
- 1 (10-oz.) pkg. frozen chopped spinach, thawed
- 1/4 cup (1 oz.) freshly grated Parmesan cheese
- 3/4 cup crème fraîche or buttermilk
- 3 eggs

SAUCE
- 1 lb. tomatoes, peeled
- 2 teaspoons finely minced fresh ginger
- 1/4 teaspoon salt

❶ Heat oven to 350°F. Butter 6 (6-oz.) custard cups or timbale molds.

❷ Melt butter in medium skillet over medium heat. Add onion, garlic and ginger; sauté 5 to 8 minutes or until browned. Add tomato sauce, coriander, cumin, red pepper, salt and turmeric. Simmer, covered, about 5 minutes or until a film of oil forms on sauce. Squeeze spinach to remove excess moisture; add to tomato sauce. Simmer, covered, 10 minutes. Remove from heat; cool.

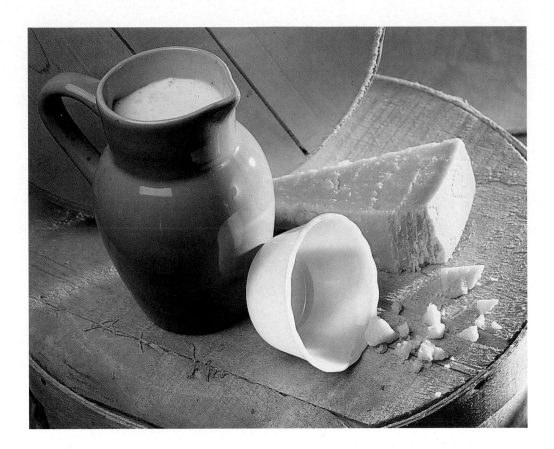

③ In food processor, puree spinach mixture. Add cheese; pulse to combine. Add crème fraîche and eggs; puree until smooth.

④ Divide mixture evenly among custard cups. Place in large shallow pan; add enough boiling water to pan to come halfway up sides of molds. Bake about 30 minutes or until spinach just begins to pull away from edges of molds.

⑤ Meanwhile, puree tomatoes, ginger and salt in food processor to form a slightly chunky sauce. Place in small saucepan; simmer over low heat just until hot.

⑥ Unmold timbales; serve with tomato sauce.

6 servings.
Preparation time: 25 minutes. Ready to serve: 1 hour, 10 minutes.

Per serving: 195 calories, 15.5 g total fat (8.5 g saturated fat), 150 mg cholesterol, 435 mg sodium, 2 g fiber.

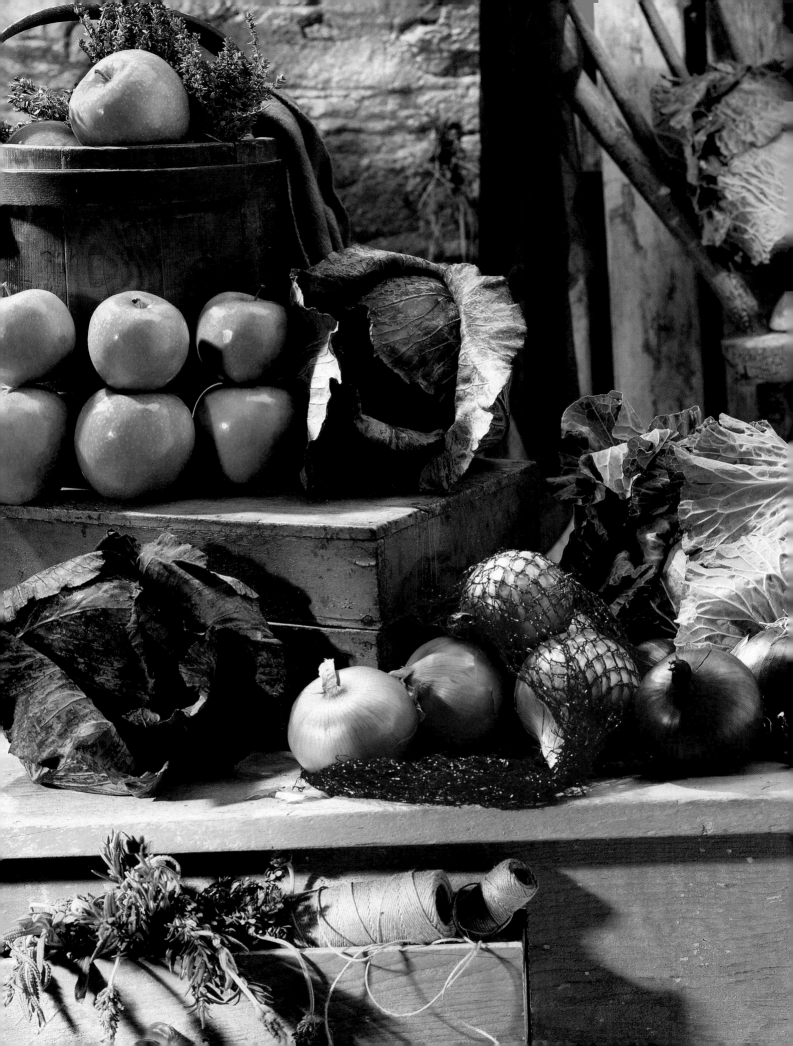

RED CABBAGE WITH APPLES AND ALLSPICE

Vinegar helps the red cabbage keep its color while cooking, as well as adding a pleasant tartness.

2 tablespoons vegetable oil
1 large onion, chopped
1 teaspoon minced garlic
1 small head red cabbage (about 1 1/2 lb.), shredded
1 cup apple cider
2 tablespoons apple cider vinegar
3/4 teaspoon dried thyme
1/4 teaspoon ground allspice
2 medium apples (such as Granny Smith or Golden Delicious), peeled, cut into 1/2-inch pieces
1/4 teaspoon salt
1/8 teaspoon freshly ground pepper

1 Heat oil in nonreactive Dutch oven or large pot over medium heat until hot. Add onion and garlic; sauté 4 to 5 minutes or until tender. Add cabbage, apple cider, cider vinegar, thyme and allspice; mix well. Reduce heat to low; cook, covered, 15 minutes, stirring occasionally.

2 Add apples; cover and cook an additional 10 minutes. Uncover; increase heat to medium. Cook an additional 10 to 15 minutes or until most liquid evaporates, stirring frequently. Season with salt and pepper. (Cabbage should have a slight peppery heat.)

8 servings.
Preparation time: 17 minutes. Ready to serve: 52 minutes.
Per serving: 90 calories, 4 g total fat (.5 g saturated fat), 0 mg cholesterol, 85 mg sodium, 2.5 g fiber.

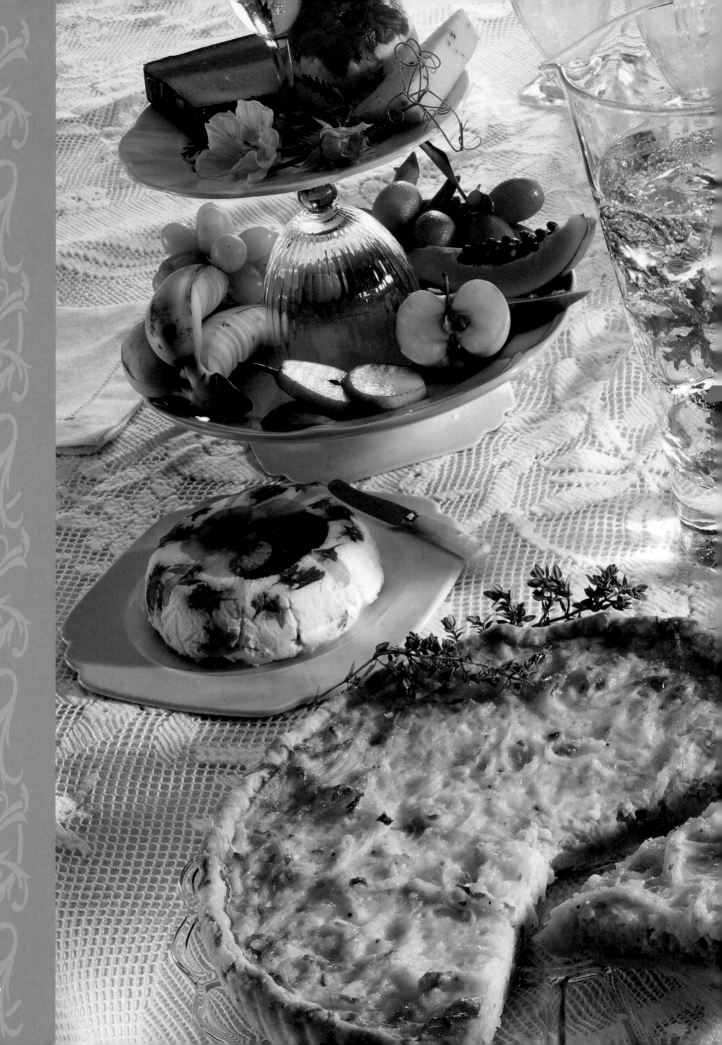

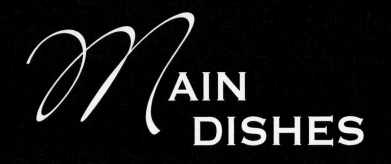

MAIN DISHES

This chapter has it all — pastas, chilies, sandwiches and brunch dishes, plus exciting flavors from regional American and ethnic cuisines. Some recipes come together quickly; others benefit from slow cooking. Pick one for a busy schedule, another for a lazy afternoon. Meat or no meat, the choice is yours with vegetarian options included for the recipes calling for meat.

Onion Tart, page 100

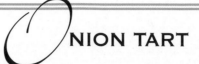NION TART

Similar to a quiche, this flavorful tart makes a wonderful luncheon dish or main course. Serve with *Winter Salad with Endive and Celery Root (page 53)* or *Spicy Pea Pod and Orange Salad (page 55).*

1   (9-inch) pie shell
2   tablespoons vegetable oil
1   tablespoon butter
4   cups thinly sliced onions
3   eggs
1/2 cup heavy cream
3/4 teaspoon salt
1/8 teaspoon freshly ground pepper
1/8 teaspoon caraway seeds
    Dash ground nutmeg
1/2 cup (2 oz.) grated Gruyère or Emmentaler cheese

1 Heat oven to 400°F. Place crust in a 9-inch tart pan with removable bottom or pie pan. Line crust with foil; fill bottom with pie weights (dried beans or rice can also be used). Bake 12 minutes or until crust is set. Remove foil and weights; return crust to oven. Bake an additional 5 minutes or until crust begins to brown. Remove from oven; cool on wire rack.

2 Heat oil and butter in large deep pot over medium-high heat until butter is melted. Add onions; sauté 4 to 5 minutes, or until slightly softened, stirring often. Reduce heat to low; cover and cook an additional 20 to 30 minutes, or until onions are very soft, stirring occasionally. Remove; cool slightly.

3 In large bowl, combine eggs, cream, salt, pepper, caraway seeds and nutmeg; mix well. Stir in onions and 1/4 cup of the cheese. Pour into pie shell. Sprinkle with remaining 1/4 cup cheese. Bake 30 to 35 minutes or until tart is puffy and golden.

4 main dish or 6 luncheon servings.
Preparation time: 20 minutes. Ready to serve: 1 hour.

Per main dish serving: 490 calories, 37 g total fat (15 g saturated fat), 215 mg cholesterol, 755 mg sodium, 2.5 g fiber.

SPAGHETTI SQUASH PUTTANESCA

Pasta puttanesca is a classic Italian dish. Using spaghetti squash instead of the more familiar noodles makes this flavorful entrée even more colorful.

1 (2½- to 3-lb.) spaghetti squash
1 tablespoon olive oil
1 tablespoon minced garlic
2 lb. tomatoes, peeled, cut into 1-inch chunks
1 (2.5-oz.) jar pitted Spanish green olives, drained, coarsely chopped
2 tablespoons capers
¼ teaspoon crushed red pepper flakes
¼ teaspoon salt

❶ Heat oven to 375°F. Place squash in shallow baking pan; prick several times with tip of knife. Bake 1 hour or until outer skin yields when pressed.

❷ Meanwhile, heat oil in large skillet over medium-high heat until hot. Add garlic; sauté 1 to 2 minutes or until fragrant and golden. Add tomatoes; cook 10 minutes. Add olives, capers, red pepper flakes and salt; cook an additional 10 minutes or until mixture thickens.

❸ Remove squash from oven; halve and remove seeds. Using spoon, remove flesh; separate into spaghetti-like strings. Place on large platter. Top with sauce.

4 servings.
Preparation time: 20 minutes. Ready to serve: 1 hour, 15 minutes.
Per serving: 165 calories, 6 g total fat (1 g saturated fat), 0 mg cholesterol, 550 mg sodium, 6 g fiber.

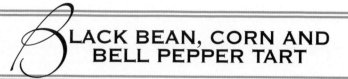BLACK BEAN, CORN AND BELL PEPPER TART

The cornmeal crust is a take-off on a Mexican tamale filling. To make this colorful dish even spicier, leave the seeds in the jalapeño before chopping.

CRUST

1½	teaspoons chili powder
1	teaspoon baking powder
1	teaspoon cumin
¾	teaspoon salt
2	tablespoons vegetable oil
1¼	cups cornmeal
1	cup boiling water
1	egg

FILLING

1	(15-oz.) can black beans, rinsed, drained
1½	cups cooked corn
1	red bell pepper, diced
½	cup chopped green onions
½	cup coarsely chopped cilantro
1	large jalapeño pepper, seeded, minced
¼	teaspoon salt
⅛	teaspoon freshly ground pepper
1½	cups shredded cheddar and mozzarella cheese blend

GARNISH

1	cup salsa

❶ Heat oven to 400°F. Grease 10-inch springform pan or pie plate with nonstick cooking spray. In medium bowl, combine chili powder, baking powder, cumin and salt; mix well. Stir in oil. Mix in cornmeal until evenly coated. Stir in water; let sit several minutes. Beat in egg. Press cornmeal mixture over bottom and ½ inch up sides of springform pan.

❷ In another medium bowl, combine all filling ingredients except ½ cup of the cheese; mix well. Spoon into crust, pressing down slightly. Sprinkle with remaining ½ cup cheese. Bake 30 minutes or until heated through and cheese is melted. Remove sides of springform pan. Serve with salsa.

6 servings.
Preparation time: 20 minutes. Ready to serve: 50 minutes.

Per serving: 380 calories, 14 g total fat (5.5 g saturated fat), 60 mg cholesterol, 880 mg sodium, 8 g fiber.

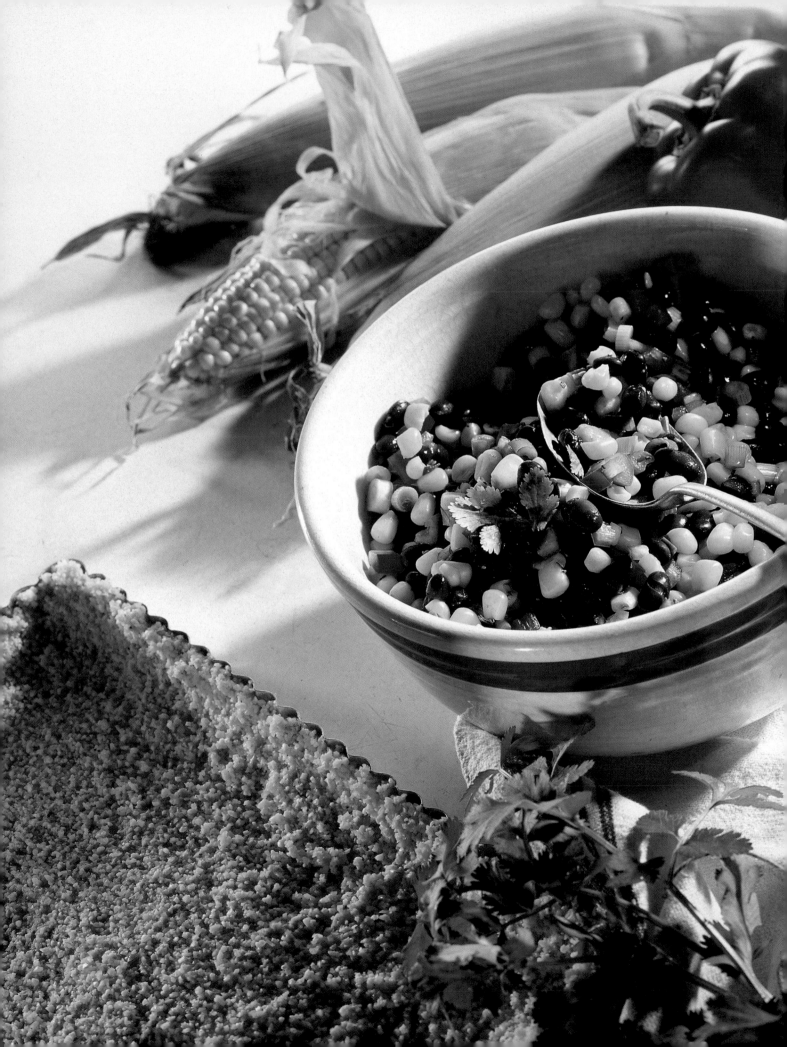

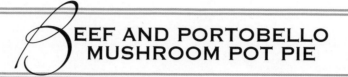

BEEF AND PORTOBELLO MUSHROOM POT PIE

Use Rich Vegetable Stock *(page 61) for the canned beef broth and add* 1/2 *teaspoon salt. The mashed potato crust is outstanding.*

FILLING

- 2 tablespoons vegetable oil
- 1 lb. lean beef for stew, cut into 3/4-inch cubes
- 1/4 cup all-purpose flour
- 1 1/4 cups beef broth
- 1/2 cup red wine
- 3/4 teaspoon dried thyme
- 12 oz. portobello mushrooms, cut into 3/4-inch cubes
- 1 1/2 cups pearl onions, peeled, or frozen whole small onions, thawed
- 3/4 cup diced carrots
- 3/4 cup peas

CRUST

- 1 1/2 pounds russet potatoes, peeled, cut into chunks
- 1 1/2 teaspoons salt
- 1/4 cup sour cream
- 1/4 cup chopped fresh chives or green onion tops
- 1/8 teaspoon freshly ground pepper

1 Heat oil in nonreactive Dutch oven or large pot over medium-high heat. Add beef in batches; cook until brown. Sprinkle with flour, stir to coat. Add broth, wine and thyme; stir, scraping bottom to remove any brown bits. Add mushrooms and onions. Bring to a boil; reduce heat to low and maintain a gentle boil. Cook 1 1/2 hours. (Mixture should be thick and reduced to about one-third of original volume.) Add carrots during last 30 minutes of cooking; add peas during last 10 minutes of cooking.

2 Meanwhile, place potatoes in large saucepan; add enough water to cover. Add 1 teaspoon of the salt. Bring to a boil over medium heat; cook 20 to 25 minutes or until potatoes are tender. Drain, reserving cooking water. Put potatoes in large bowl; mash. Stir in sour cream and enough cooking water to make potatoes fluffy and smooth. Stir in chives, remaining 1/2 teaspoon salt and pepper.

3 Heat broiler. When beef mixture is tender, transfer to deep 9-inch pie plate. Top with potatoes; broil 5 minutes or until browned.

6 servings.

Preparation time: 50 minutes. Ready to serve: 2 hours, 25 minutes.

Per serving: 365 calories, 15.5 g total fat (5 g saturated fat), 55 mg cholesterol, 675 mg sodium, 4.5 g fiber.

CAULIFLOWER AND GARBANZO BEAN TAGINE

Tagine is Morocco's version of stew. Serve this dish with Spicy Pea Pod and Orange Salad *(page 55).*

1	tablespoon vegetable oil
1	large onion, chopped
2	teaspoons paprika
1	teaspoon ground cumin
1/2	teaspoon ground ginger
1/4	teaspoon salt
1/8	teaspoon cayenne
2	cups *Light Vegetable Stock* (page 60) or water
2	tablespoons lemon juice
1	(2- to 2 1/2-lb.) cauliflower, florets only
1	stick cinnamon
1	(15-oz.) can garbanzo beans, rinsed, drained
1	red bell pepper, seeded, cut into 1/2-inch pieces
2	tablespoons chopped fresh cilantro

❶ Heat oil in nonreactive Dutch oven or large pot over medium-high heat until hot. Add onion; sauté 5 to 7 minutes or until lightly browned. Stir in paprika, cumin, ginger, salt and cayenne; cook 30 to 60 minutes or until fragrant. Stir in stock and lemon juice; add cauliflower and cinnamon stick. Bring to boil; reduce heat to medium-low. Cook, covered, 10 minutes.

❷ Add beans and bell pepper; reduce heat to low. Cook, covered, an additional 10 minutes. Remove cinnamon stick; sprinkle with cilantro. Serve over cooked couscous, if desired.

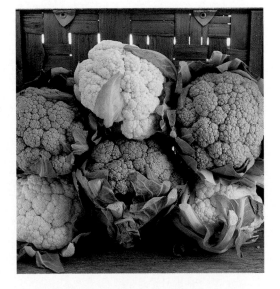

6 servings.
Preparation time: 15 minutes.
Ready to serve: 50 minutes.

Per serving: 140 calories, 4 g total fat (.5 g saturated fat), 0 mg cholesterol, 240 mg sodium, 5.5 g fiber.

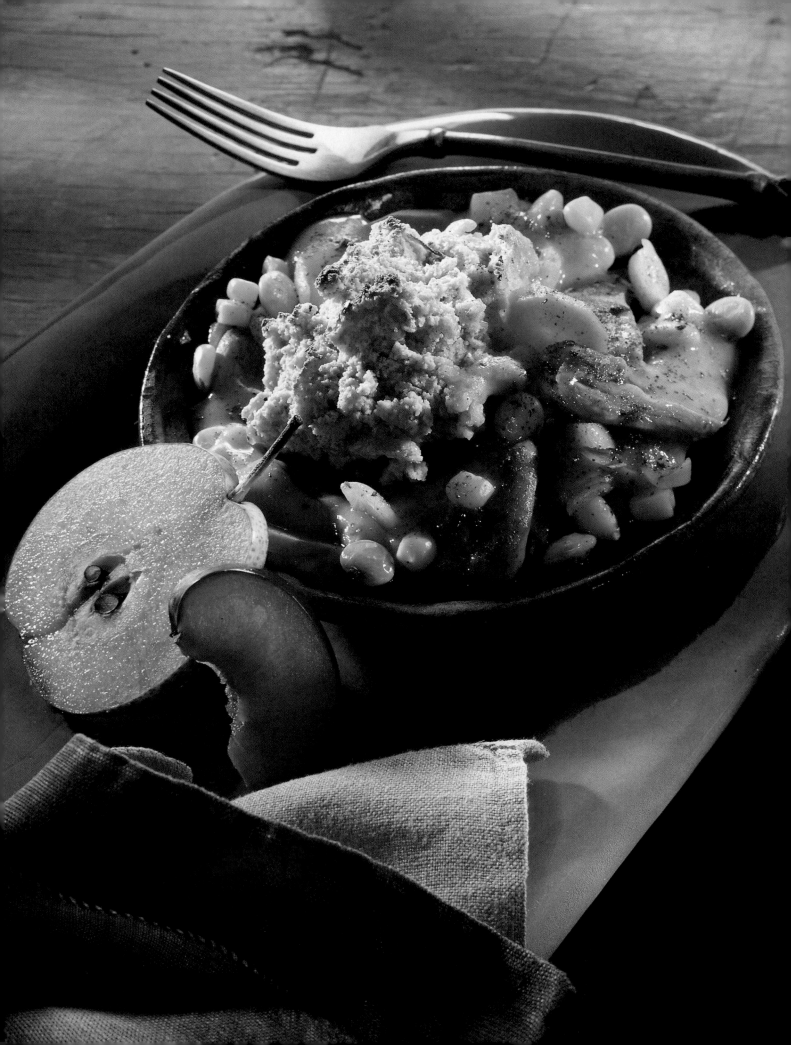

CHICKEN, VEGETABLE AND CORNBREAD COBBLER

The Cajun seasoning adds a spicy kick to this savory cobbler. To make this dish vegetarian, substitute one (15-oz.) can red or kidney beans, rinsed and drained, for the chicken.

3	tablespoons vegetable oil
1	lb. boneless skinless chicken thighs, cubed
1	large onion, chopped
1/3	cup all-purpose flour
2 to 3	teaspoons Cajun seasoning
1¾	cups water or *Light Vegetable Stock* (page 60)
1½	cups corn
1½	cups lima beans
2	medium carrots, peeled, sliced
1	(8.5-oz.) box cornbread mix
1/3	cup milk
1	egg

❶ Heat oven to 400°F. Heat oil in large skillet over medium-high heat until hot. Add chicken and onion; sauté 3 to 4 minutes or until tender. Sprinkle with flour and Cajun seasoning; stir to combine. Whisk in water. Bring to a boil; add corn, beans and carrots. Bring to a simmer; reduce heat to low. Cook, covered, 15 minutes, stirring occasionally. Pour into 8 x 12-inch (2-quart) baking dish.

❷ In medium bowl, combine cornbread mix, milk and egg; mix well. Drop by spoonfuls over surface of chicken mixture; spread gently to cover, leaving ½-inch border around edge. Bake 20 minutes or until cornbread is golden and filling is bubbly.

6 servings.
Preparation time: 16 minutes. Ready to serve: 55 minutes.
Per serving: 480 calories, 21 g total fat (6 g saturated fat), 90 mg cholesterol, 595 mg sodium, 7 g fiber.

CHORIZO CHILI

Chorizo is a type of sausage found in Mexican and southwestern cooking. Feel free to substitute a spicy Italian sausage if unavailable. Use canned tomatoes for convenience or when fresh ones are out of season. To make this dish vegetarian, substitute one (15-oz.) can of pinto or garbanzo beans for the chorizo, and add a chopped chipotle chile or jalepeño pepper to liven up the seasoning.

1	tablespoon vegetable oil
1/2	lb. chorizo or other spicy sausage, sliced
1	large onion, chopped (1 cup)
1	green pepper, chopped
1	tablespoon minced garlic
1	(28-oz.) can diced tomatoes, undrained, or 2 pounds chopped fresh tomatoes
1	(15-oz.) can kidney beans, rinsed, drained
1	(14.5-oz) can beef broth
2	tablespoons chili powder
1	teaspoon ground cumin
1/2	teaspoon dried oregano
1/8	teaspoon cayenne
1	cup corn

❶ Heat nonreactive Dutch oven or large pot over medium-high heat. Add oil; heat until hot. Add chorizo; sauté 2 to 3 minutes or until chorizo begins to brown. Add onion, green pepper and garlic; sauté 3 to 4 minutes or until vegetables begin to soften. Add tomatoes, beans, broth, chili powder, cumin and oregano; mix well. Bring to a boil; reduce heat to low. Simmer, partially covered, 20 minutes. Add corn; cook an additional 10 minutes.

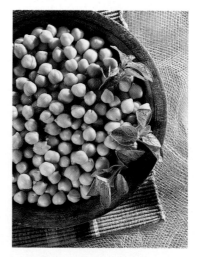

4 to 6 servings.
Preparation time: 15 minutes.
Ready to serve: 40 minutes.

Per serving: 475 calories, 27 g total fat (9 g saturated fat), 50 mg cholesterol, 1755 mg sodium, 9 g fiber.

$\mathcal{I}$NDIAN ROOT VEGETABLE CURRY

Curries are synonymous with India and the word originates from the Indian word "karhi," meaning sauce. In other parts of the world, curries are often erroneously considered a spice or a blend of spices, a concept that is non-existent in India. Versions of this root vegetable stew are found all over southern India, and this curry derives its flavors from chiles, coconut and cilantro. If you can't find unsweetened coconut, substitute the sweetened kind but rinse it thoroughly under cold water first, then pat it dry.

1 1/2	cups water
1	medium white or red potato, peeled, cut into 1/2-inch cubes
1	medium sweet potato, peeled, cut into 1/2-inch cubes
1	medium carrot, peeled, cut into 1/2-inch cubes
1/2	cup chopped red onion
1	cup freshly grated coconut (or 1/2 cup dried unsweetened coconut, shredded)
3 to 4	fresh serrano chilies
1/2	cup fresh cilantro
1	medium tomato, cut into 1/2-inch cubes
1	cup peas
1	teaspoon vegetable oil
1	teaspoon ground cumin
1	teaspoon salt

❶ In medium saucepan, bring water, white potato, sweet potato, carrot and onion to a boil over medium-high heat. Reduce heat to low; simmer, covered, 6 to 8 minutes or until vegetables are al dente.

❷ Meanwhile, place coconut, chiles, and cilantro in food processor; process until chiles and cilantro are finely minced. Add coconut mixture, tomato and peas to potato mixture; mix well. Simmer, uncovered, 4 to 6 minutes or until peas are cooked through.

❸ Heat oil in small skillet over medium-high heat until hot; add cumin seed. Cook 15 to 20 seconds. Add oil mixture to vegetable mixture; season with salt. Mix well. Serve with cooked rice, if desired.

6 servings.
Preparation time: 18 minutes. Ready to serve: 40 minutes.
Per serving: 135 calories, 5.5 g total fat (4 g saturated fat), 0 mg cholesterol, 425 mg sodium, 4.5 g fiber.

FOUR SEASONS PIZZA

This is a classic Italian pizza with the four sections representing the four seasons. Use this recipe as a base for any vegetable topping you choose.

CRUST
- 1 cup lukewarm water (105°F to 115°F)
- 1 (1/4-oz.) pkg. active dry yeast
- 3 cups all-purpose flour
- 2 teaspoons sugar
- 1/2 teaspoon salt
- 1 tablespoon olive oil

TOPPING
- 1 (8-oz.) can tomato sauce
- 4 oz. white mushrooms, thinly sliced
- 1 tablespoon olive oil
- 1/2 green bell pepper, thinly sliced
- 1 (6.5-oz.) jar marinated artichoke hearts, drained, coarsely chopped
- 2 to 3 plum tomatoes, thinly sliced
- 2 cups (8 oz.) shredded mozzarella cheese

❶ Heat oven to 450°F. Lightly spray 2 baking sheets or 2 (14-inch) pizza pans with nonstick cooking spray. Combine water and yeast in small bowl; let sit 5 minutes. In large bowl, combine 2 1/2 cups of the flour, sugar and salt; mix well. Add yeast mixture and oil to flour mixture; stir to make a soft dough. Dust work surface with remaining 1/2 cup flour. Turn dough out onto floured surface, knead until smooth dough forms, adding additional flour if needed to prevent sticking.

❷ Divide dough in half; shape each half into disk. Roll each disk into a 14-inch round. Place on baking sheets; spread each with half of tomato sauce. In medium bowl, toss mushrooms with 1 tablespoon oil. Cover 1/4 of each pizza with mushrooms, 1/4 with bell pepper, 1/4 with artichoke hearts and 1/4 with tomatoes. Sprinkle each pizza with 1 cup of the cheese. Bake 10 to 12 minutes or until browned and crisp.

2 (14-inch) pizzas, 8 slices each.
Preparation time: 25 minutes. Ready to serve: 43 minutes.
Per slice: 420 calories, 12.5 g total fat (5 g saturated fat), 20 mg cholesterol, 705 mg sodium, 4 g fiber.

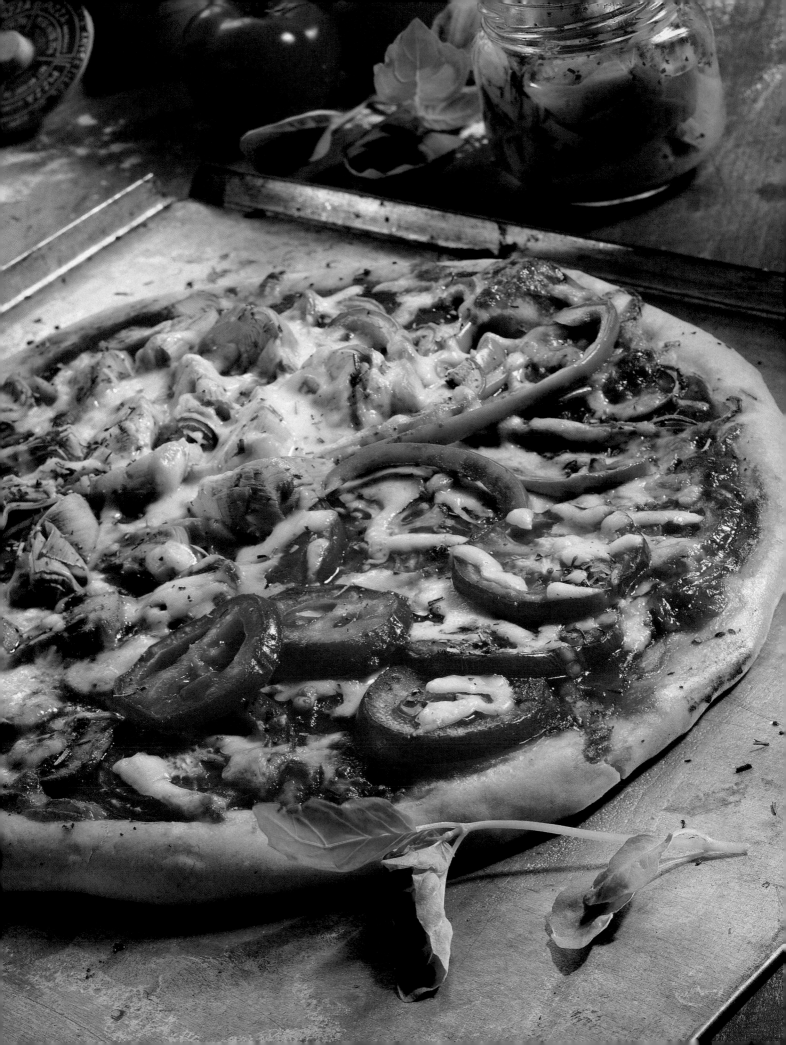

SQUASH RAVIOLI WITH RED PEPPER SAUCE

Cooked squash often has excess moisture. Place the squash in a fine strainer for 15 minutes before use, gently turning from time to time, to allow it to drain.

SAUCE

2	red bell peppers, halved
1/2	cup reduced-sodium chicken broth or 1/3 cup *Light Vegetable Stock* (page 60)
2	tablespoons sour cream
1/4	teaspoon salt

FILLING

1	cup drained cooked squash (such as butternut)*
3/4	cup (3 oz.) freshly grated Parmesan cheese
1/4	cup dry bread crumbs
1	egg
3/4	teaspoon dried sage
1/8	teaspoon freshly ground pepper

PASTA**

1 1/3 to 1 1/2	cups all-purpose flour
2	teaspoons salt
2	eggs

1 Heat broiler. Line shallow baking pan with foil. Place bell peppers on pan skin side up; broil 4 to 6 inches from heat 7 to 10 minutes or until blackened. Remove. Place in bowl; cover. Let sit 5 minutes. Remove charred skin and seeds. Place bell peppers and broth in food processor or blender; puree. Set aside.

2 In medium bowl, combine squash, cheese, breadcrumbs, egg, sage and pepper. Set aside.

3 In food processor, combine 1/3 cup of the flour and 2 teaspoons of the salt. With motor running, add eggs one at a time; process until mixture forms small grains of pasta. (Dough should not be sticky. Add additional flour if necessary.) Pat dough into ball; divide into 4 pieces.

4 Work with one piece of dough at a time, keeping remaining dough covered with towel. Roll dough into cylinder; flatten to about 1/2-inch thickness. Using hand-cranked pasta machine, feed dough through using widest setting. Feed dough through again using next to the lowest setting, dusting as necessary with small amount of flour to prevent dough from sticking. On very lightly floured surface, trim dough to 4-inch-wide strip. Place ¹/₂ tablespoon squash filling every 2 inches along right side of strip until there are 12 circles of filling. Using finger dipped in water, dampen dough around filling. Fold dough in half lengthwise; press around filling to seal. Cut into 12 squares trimming away excess dough. Set aside on very lightly floured surface. Repeat with remaining dough.

⑤ Bring large pot of water to a boil. Add remaining 2 teaspoons salt. Add ravioli; cook 3 to 4 minutes. Drain.

⑥ While ravioli are cooking, place bell pepper mixture in medium saucepan. Bring to a boil over medium-low heat. Remove from heat; stir in sour cream and 2 teaspoons salt. Reserve ¹/₄ cup sauce. Divide remaining sauce among 4 plates, creating ring of sauce on each plate. Place drained ravioli in center of rings. Garnish center of each with 1 tablespoon of sauce.

TIP *To cook squash, heat oven to 375°F. Line baking sheet with foil; lightly grease. Cut squash in half lengthwise; place on baking sheet. Bake 1 hour or until tender. Scoop flesh from shell; freeze excess squash in plastic freezer bag for another use.

TIP **Gyoza or wonton skins can be substituted for freshly made pasta. Use 48 skins. Place 1 tablespoon of filling in center of each of 24 skins. Dampen edge of each with water; top with remaining skins. Press to seal. Cook in boiling salted water 2 to 3 minutes.

4 servings.
Preparation time: 42 minutes. Ready to serve: 2 hours.

Per serving: 385 calories, 12.5 g total fat (6.5 g saturated fat), 180 mg cholesterol, 1875 mg sodium, 3 g fiber.

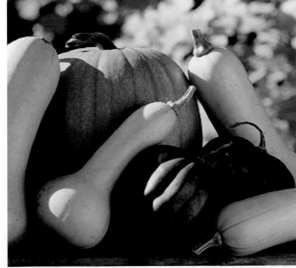

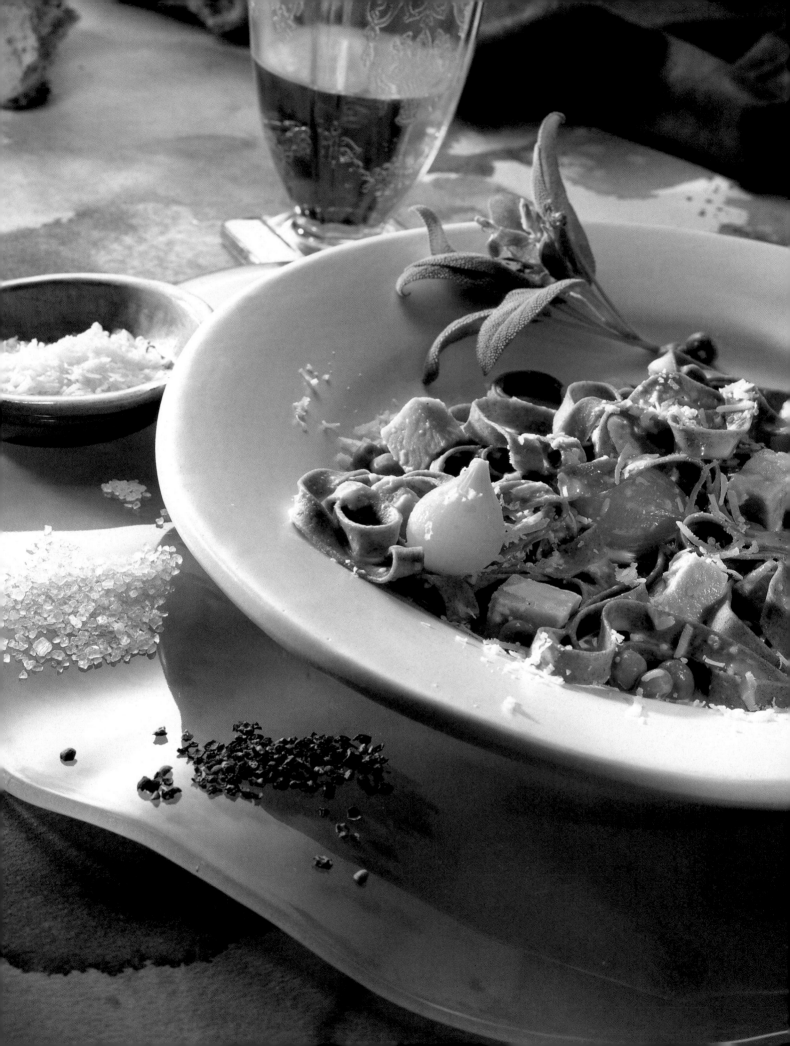

PEAS, PEARL ONIONS, SMOKED TURKEY AND PARMESAN PASTA

Frozen vegetables are the first choice to make this dish quickly. To make a vegetarian version, substitute another vegetable for the turkey (perhaps asparagus or carrots) and grate a smoked cheese (such as provolone) over the finished dish.

16 to 20 frozen small whole onions (or skinned fresh pearl onions)
1 cup reduced-sodium chicken broth
1 cup frozen or fresh shelled peas
1/2 lb. smoked turkey, cut into 1/2-inch pieces
1/2 cup whipping cream
1/8 teaspoon freshly ground pepper
1 (9-oz.) pkg. fresh or dried fettuccini
1/4 cup (1 oz.) freshly grated Parmesan cheese

① In large skillet over medium-low heat, cook onions and broth, covered, 10 minutes or until onions are tender. Uncover; add peas, turkey, cream and pepper. Increase heat to medium-high; bring to boil. Cook 5 to 8 minutes or until peas are tender and sauce has reduced slightly.

② Meanwhile, cook fettuccine according to package directions. Drain. Place sauce in large shallow bowl. Stir in 2 tablespoons of the cheese. Add fettuccine; toss to coat. Sprinkle with remaining 2 tablespoons cheese; toss. Serve with additional cheese if desired.

4 servings.
Preparation time: 5 minutes. Ready to serve: 20 minutes.

Per serving: 460 calories, 17 g total fat (8.5 g saturated fat), 12.5 mg cholesterol, 1135 mg sodium, 4.5 g fiber.

TABBOULEH FETA POCKETS

Add bits of cooked lamb or chicken to this sandwich, if desired, or serve the filling as a salad accompaniment.

1	cup water
½	cup bulgur
1	medium tomato, chopped
½	medium cucumber, peeled, chopped (about ½ cup)
2	oz. feta cheese, crumbled (about ½ cup)
¼	cup chopped green onions
¼	cup chopped fresh mint
¼	cup chopped fresh parsley
2	tablespoons sliced ripe olives
2	tablespoons lemon juice
2	tablespoons extra-virgin olive oil
¼	teaspoon salt
⅛	teaspoon freshly ground pepper
3	pitas

1 In small saucepan over medium heat, bring water and bulgur to a boil. Reduce heat to low; simmer 5 minutes. Remove from heat; cover. Let sit 5 minutes; cool.

2 In medium bowl, combine bulgur, tomato, cucumber, cheese, onions, mint, parsley and olives. In small bowl, combine lemon juice, oil, salt and pepper. Toss with bulgur mixture. Refrigerate, covered, until ready to serve.

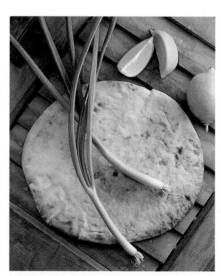

3 Cut pitas in half; fill pockets evenly with mixture.

6 servings.
Preparation time: 15 minutes.
Ready to serve: 30 minutes.

Per serving: 180 calories, 7.5 g total fat (2 g saturated fat), 10 mg cholesterol, 355 mg sodium, 3.5 g fiber.

$\mathcal{V}$EGETARIAN GUMBO

Making a roux involves cooking butter or oil and flour together and is a common technique in recipes from France and Louisiana. What sets the Louisiana technique apart is the custom of browning the roux. This adds a rich and nutty flavor to the finished dish.

1/4 cup vegetable oil
1/4 cup all-purpose flour
1 large onion, chopped
1 large green bell pepper, chopped
1 1/2 teaspoons minced garlic
1 lb. tomatoes, coarsely chopped
2 cups water
2 cups sliced okra
1 (15-oz.) can kidney beans, rinsed, drained
2 teaspoons Cajun seasoning
1/2 teaspoon salt
1/8 teaspoon freshly ground black pepper
1 bunch collard greens (about 1/2-lb.), stemmed, coarsely chopped

❶ Heat oil in nonreactive Dutch oven or large pot over medium-high heat until hot. Stir in flour; cook about 5 minutes or until flour turns to a medium brown, stirring constantly. Stir in onion, bell pepper and garlic; cook 3 to 4 minutes or until vegetables begin to soften, stirring constantly.

❷ Add tomatoes, water, okra, beans, Cajun seasoning, salt and pepper; stir to combine. Reduce heat to low; cook, partially covered, 30 minutes. Add collard greens; cook an additional 10 minutes. Serve over cooked rice, if desired.

6 (1-cup) servings.
Preparation time: 25 minutes. Ready to serve: 1 hour, 5 minutes.
Per serving: 200 calories, 10 g total fat (1.5 g saturated fat), 0 mg cholesterol, 425 mg sodium, 5.5 g fiber.

TOMATO-OLIVE RAGOUT WITH POLENTA

To peel tomatoes, bring a large pot of water to a boil. Drop tomatoes in water for approximately one minute. Plunge into cold water. Skins should come off easily with a sharp knife. Kalamata olives are dark, Greek olives packed in brine. If possible, buy them already pitted. Otherwise, press down on the olive with the flat side of a large knife blade; this crushes the olive and loosens the pit.

RAGOUT

- 2 tablespoons olive oil
- 1 large onion, sliced
- 1 medium bulb fennel, fronds removed, sliced
- 1 tablespoon minced garlic
- 8 oz. crimini mushrooms, sliced
- 2 lb. tomatoes, peeled, cut into 1-inch pieces
- 1/2 cup pitted Kalamata olives
- 1/4 teaspoon salt

POLENTA

- 3 cups water
- 1/2 teaspoon salt
- 1/2 teaspoon dried thyme
- 3/4 cup polenta style cornmeal

❶ Heat oil in nonreactive Dutch oven or large pot over medium heat until hot. Add onion and fennel; sauté 4 to 5 minutes or until onion and fennel begin to soften. Add garlic; cook 1 minute. Add mushrooms; sauté an additional 4 to 5 minutes. Add tomatoes, olives and 1/4 teaspoon salt; cook 20 to 25 minutes or until tomatoes have reduced and ragout has thickened, stirring occasionally.

❷ Lightly grease 8-inch square pan. In medium saucepan, bring water, 1/2 teaspoon salt and thyme to a boil over medium heat. Slowly whisk in cornmeal. Reduce heat to low; cook 5 to 10 minutes or until mixture thickens and polenta begins to pull away from sides of pan, stirring constantly. Pour into pan; let sit until firm.

❸ Cut into fourths; cut each fourth into triangles. Place two triangles on each plate. Top with 1/4 of ragout.

4 servings.
Preparation time: 35 minutes. Ready to serve: 45 minutes.
Per serving: 270 calories, 10.5 g total fat (1.5 g saturated fat), 0 mg cholesterol, 650 mg sodium, 7.5 g fiber.

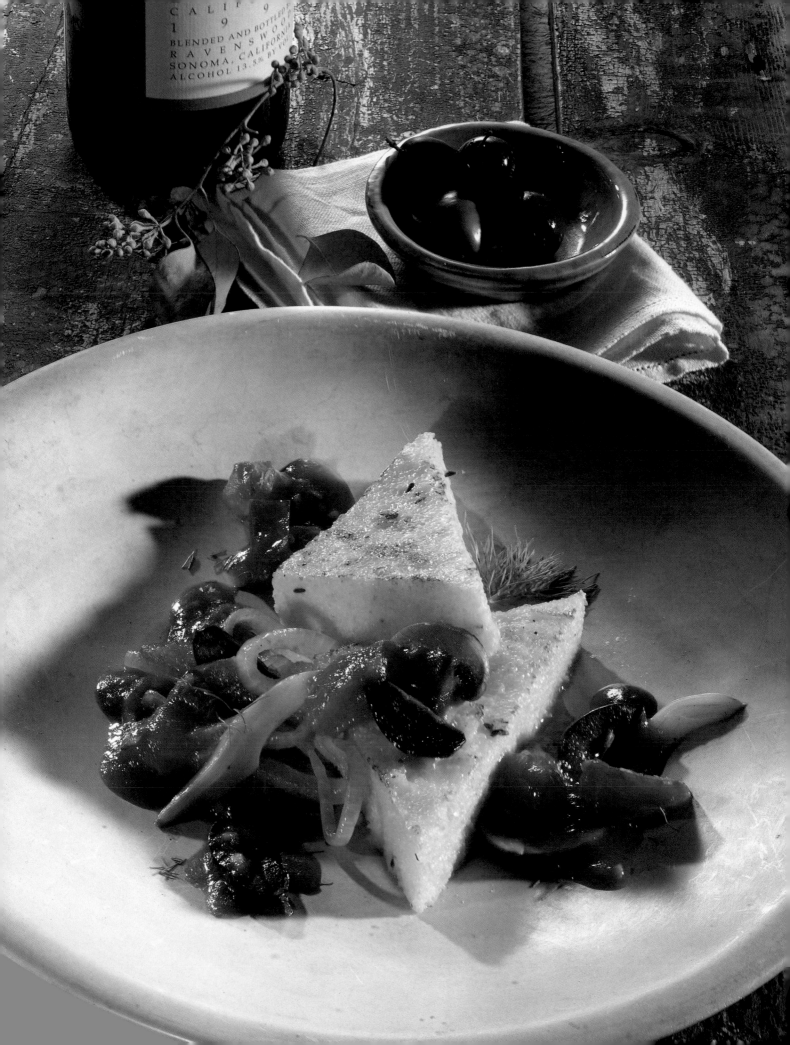

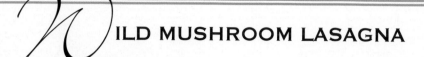ILD MUSHROOM LASAGNA

Cooking the mushrooms with the soaking liquid from the dried mushrooms intensifies the porcini flavor.

- 1 (1-oz.) pkg. dried porcini mushrooms
- 1 cup very hot water
- 1 tablespoon vegetable oil
- 1 small onion, chopped
- 1 tablespoon minced garlic
- 1 lb. assorted fresh mushrooms (such as white, crimini and chanterelle), chopped
- 3/4 cup dry red wine
- 1/4 teaspoon dried thyme
- 1/2 teaspoon salt
- 1/4 teaspoon freshly ground pepper
- 3 tablespoons water
- 5 teaspoons all-purpose flour
- 1 (15-oz.) container ricotta cheese or dry curd cottage cheese
- 1/4 cup (1-oz.) freshly grated Parmesan cheese
- 1/4 cup chopped chives or green onion tops
- 1 egg
- 6 cooked lasagna noodles
- 4 oz. grated mozzarella cheese (about 1 cup)

1 Soak dried mushrooms in hot water 30 minutes; remove mushrooms. Strain soaking liquid through coffee filter; reserve liquid. Chop mushrooms; set aside.

2 Heat oven to 350°F. Heat oil in large skillet over medium-high heat until hot. Add onion; sauté 3 to 4 minutes or until softened. Add garlic; sauté 1 minute or until fragrant. Add 1 lb. mushrooms; sauté 5 to 8 minutes or until tender. Add wine, porcini mushrooms, reserved soaking liquid, thyme, 1/4 teaspoon of the salt and 1/8 teaspoon of the pepper. Reduce heat to medium-low; simmer 10 minutes.

3 In small bowl, whisk together water and flour. Whisk flour mixture into mushroom mixture; simmer 2 to 3 minutes or until slightly thickened. Meanwhile, in medium bowl, combine ricotta cheese, Parmesan cheese, chives, egg and remaining 1/4 teaspoon salt and 1/8 teaspoon pepper.

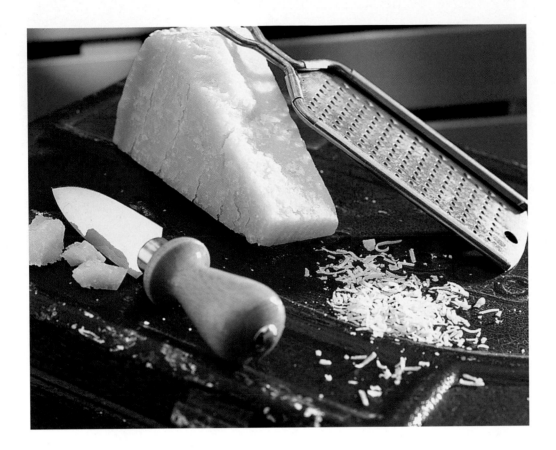

4. To assemble, spread half of mushroom mixture on bottom of 8 x 12-inch (or 9 x 13-inch) baking dish. Arrange 3 of the cooked lasagna noodles on top of mushroom mixture; spoon and spread cheese mixture over noodles. Top with 3 remaining noodles; finish topping with remaining mushroom mixture. Sprinkle top with mozzarella cheese.

5. Bake, covered, 30 to 35 minutes or until heated through and bubbly. Uncover; let sit 10 minutes before serving.

6 servings.
Preparation time: 30 minutes. Ready to serve: 1 hour, 40 minutes.

Per serving: 325 calories, 14 g total fat (7 g saturated fat), 70 mg cholesterol, 565 mg sodium, 2 g fiber.

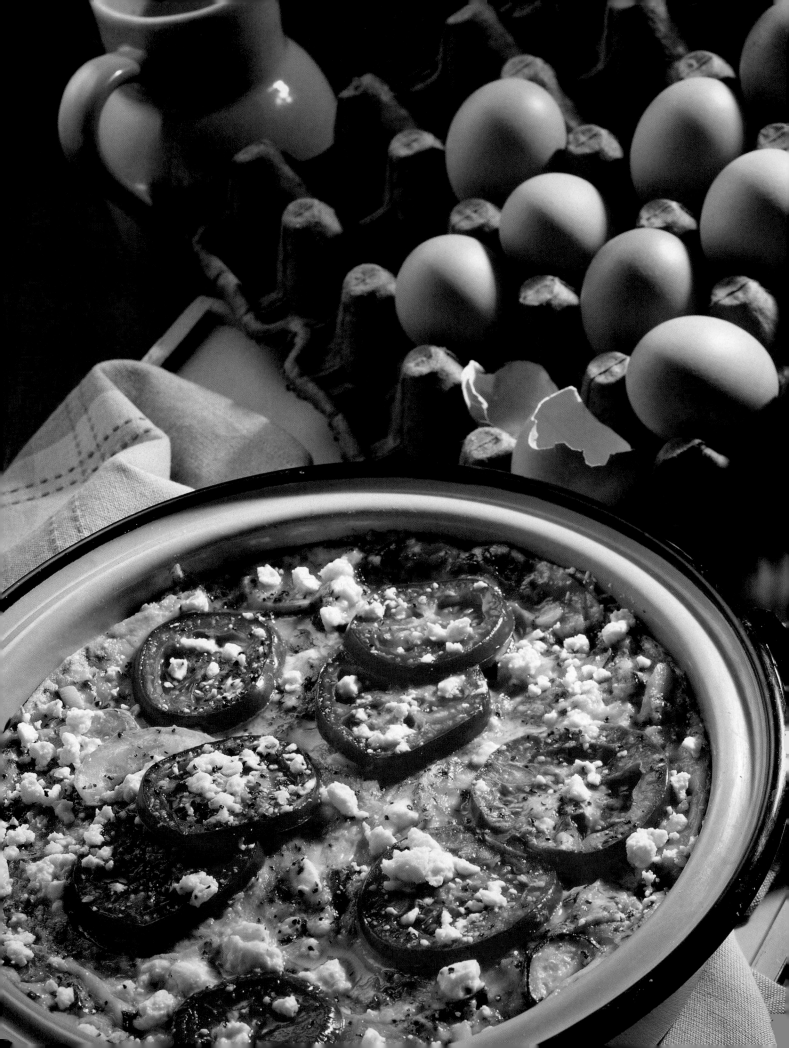

ZUCCHINI AND TOMATO FRITTATA

Serve this dish for brunch along with Frosty Marys *(page 24). Add* Corn and Barley Salad *(page 43) plus your favorite muffin to round out the menu.*

3 tablespoons olive oil
1 large onion, chopped
1 small zucchini, halved, sliced
1 small summer squash, halved, sliced
2 teaspoons minced garlic
8 eggs
3/4 teaspoon dried oregano
1/2 teaspoon dried dill weed
1/2 teaspoon salt
1/4 teaspoon freshly ground pepper
2 oz. crumbled feta cheese (about 1/2 cup)
1 medium tomato, sliced

❶ Heat oil in large nonstick skillet over medium-high heat until hot. Add onion; sauté 4 to 5 minutes or until softened. Add zucchini, squash and garlic; sauté 5 minutes or until zucchini and squash have softened.

❷ In medium bowl, combine eggs, oregano, dill weed, salt and pepper; beat well. Reduce heat to low; add egg mixture to squash mixture. Sprinkle with cheese. Cover and cook 5 minutes, pushing egg back from sides of pan. Occasionally tip pan and cut through egg mixture with spatula to allow uncooked egg to run to bottom of pan. Top with sliced tomato; continue to cook, covered, 5 to 7 minutes, occasionally pushing and tipping eggs.

❸ When egg mixture has set, slide onto serving platter.

4 servings.
Preparation time: 30 minutes. Ready to serve: 30 minutes.
Per serving: 310 calories, 23.5 g total fat (6.5 g saturated fat), 440 mg cholesterol, 580 mg sodium, 2 g fiber.

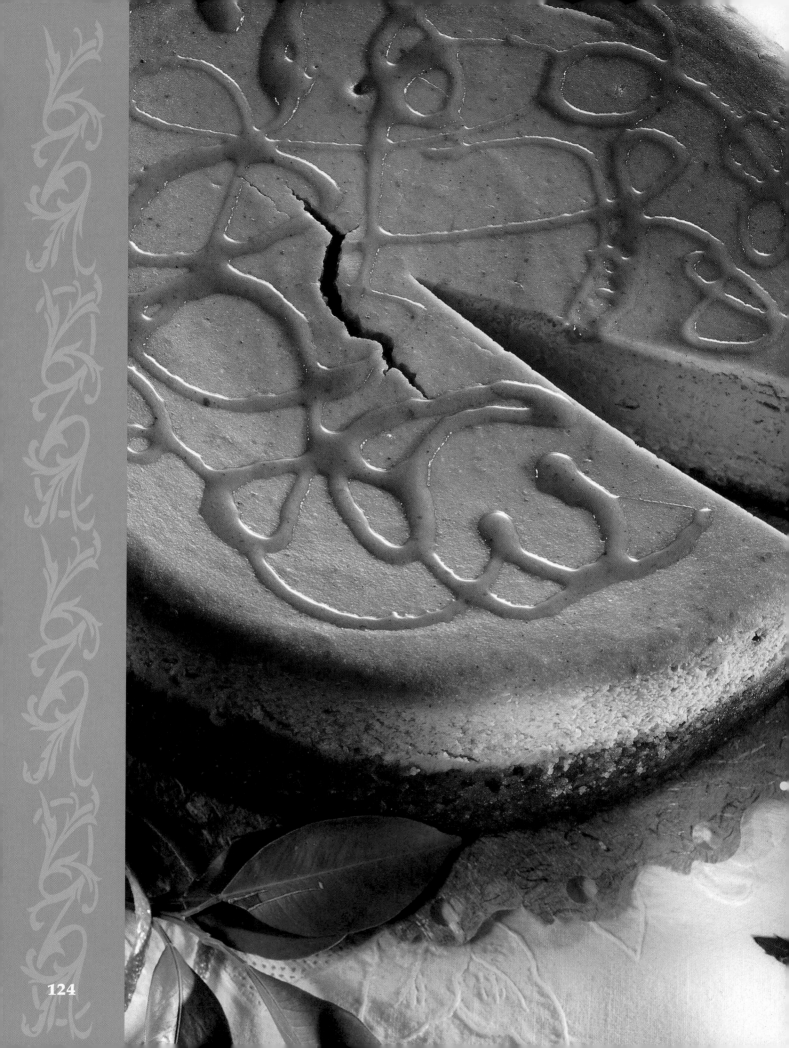

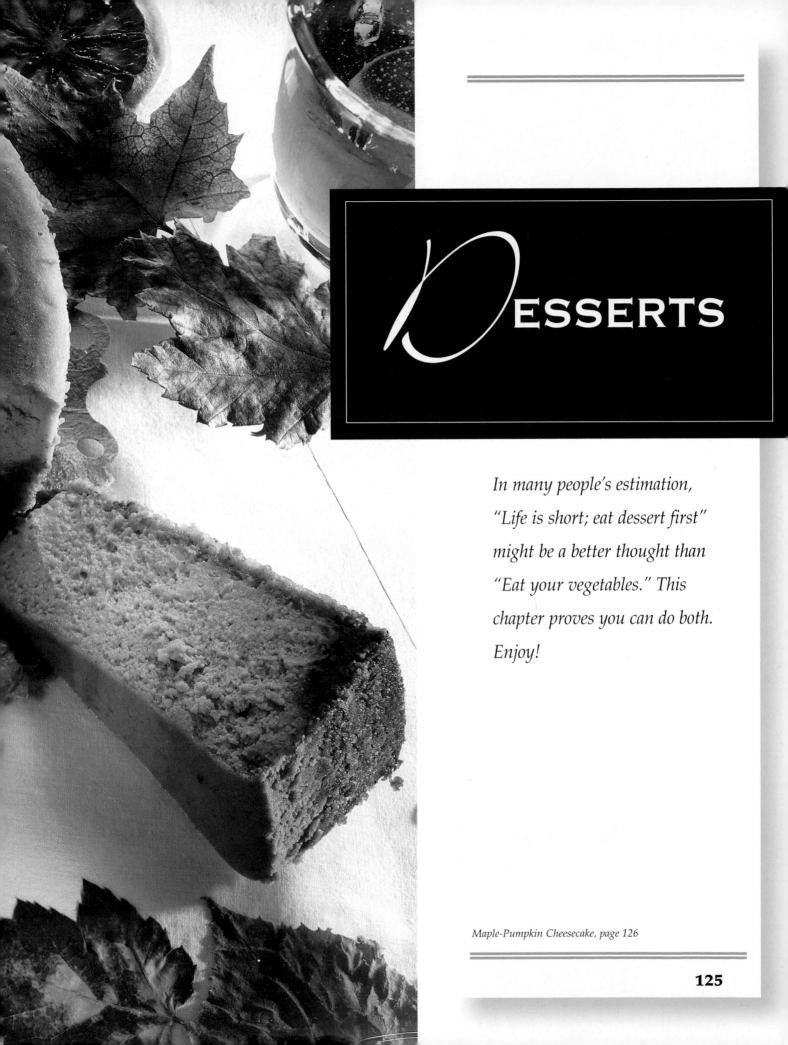

DESSERTS

In many people's estimation, "Life is short; eat dessert first" might be a better thought than "Eat your vegetables." This chapter proves you can do both. Enjoy!

Maple-Pumpkin Cheesecake, page 126

$\mathcal{M}$APLE-PUMPKIN CHEESECAKE

To save time, serve this cheesecake with purchased caramel topping or simply top with a spoonful of lightly sweetened whipped cream.

CRUST
- 3/4 cup chopped walnuts
- 3/4 cup graham cracker crumbs
- 1/4 cup sugar
- 1/4 cup butter, melted, cooled

FILLING
- 3 (8-oz.) pkg. cream cheese, softened
- 1 cup packed light brown sugar
- 4 eggs, room temperature
- 1/4 cup sugar
- 3 tablespoons all-purpose flour
- 1 1/2 teaspoons ground cinnamon
- 1/2 teaspoon ground ginger
- 1/4 teaspoon ground nutmeg
- 1 (8-oz.) container sour cream
- 3/4 teaspoon maple extract
- 2 cups cooked pumpkin* (or 1 (15-oz.) can)

TOPPING
- 3/4 cup maple syrup
- 1/2 cup packed light brown sugar
- 1/2 cup apple cider or water

❶ Heat oven to 350°F. In food processor, pulse together walnuts and graham cracker crumbs until finely ground. Add 1/4 cup sugar; pulse to combine. Add butter; pulse to combine. Pat mixture over bottom and 1 inch up sides of 10-inch springform pan. Bake 10 minutes. Remove from oven; let cool.

❷ In large bowl, beat cream cheese at medium speed until soft. Add 1 cup brown sugar; beat until very soft. Add eggs one at a time, beating only until combined after each addition. In medium bowl, whisk together 1/4 cup sugar, flour, cinnamon, ginger and nutmeg. Whisk in sour cream and maple extract. Beat sour cream mixture into cream cheese mixture at low speed just until combined. Stir in pumpkin. Pour into springform pan. Place springform pan on baking sheet; bake 55 to 65 minutes or until center is just set. (Center should be less set than edges and will move when pan is tapped.) Cool on wire rack 1 hour. Cover; refrigerate 3 to 4 hours or overnight.

❸ To make topping, place maple syrup, brown sugar and apple cider in medium saucepan. Cook over medium heat until mixture comes to a boil, stirring occasionally. Continue to boil without stirring 10 minutes or until mixture has reduced and slightly thickened. To serve, spoon sauce over cheesecake.

TIP *To cook pumpkin, halve 2¹/₂- to 3-lb. pumpkin lengthwise. Place on foil-lined shallow pan; bake at 375°F for 1 hour or until very soft. Cool. Remove seeds; scrape out flesh. Place flesh in fine strainer over small bowl 15 minutes, to allow to drain, turning occasionally.

12 servings.
Preparation time: 25 minutes. Ready to serve: 6 hours, 40 minutes.

Per serving: 580 calories, 34.5 g total fat (18.5 g saturated fat), 155 mg cholesterol, 265 mg sodium, 2 g fiber.

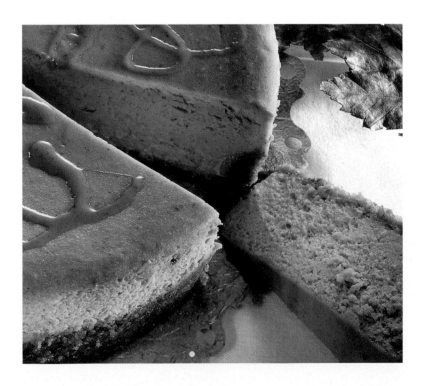

TRIPLE CHOCOLATE ZUCCHINI CAKE

Zucchini is the magic ingredient in this yummy cake. Hidden in all the chocolate, it adds moistness and body.

CAKE
- 1/4 cup milk
- 1/4 cup orange juice
- 1 tablespoon grated orange peel
- 3/4 cup butter, softened
- 2 cups sugar
- 3 eggs
- 2 1/4 cups all-purpose flour
- 1/2 cup unsweetened cocoa
- 2 teaspoons baking powder
- 1 teaspoon ground cinnamon
- 3/4 teaspoon baking soda
- 1/2 teaspoon salt
- 2 cups shredded unpeeled zucchini
- 1 cup (6 oz.) semisweet chocolate chips

GLAZE
- 3 oz. milk chocolate, chopped
- 5 teaspoons orange juice

① Heat oven to 350°F. Spray 10-inch Bundt pan with nonstick cooking spray; dust with flour. In small bowl, combine milk, orange juice and orange peel. Set aside.

② Beat butter in large bowl at medium speed until creamy. Add sugar; beat until fluffy. Add eggs one at a time, beating well after each addition.

③ In another large bowl, sift together flour, cocoa, baking powder, cinnamon, baking soda and salt. Beat half of flour mixture into butter mixture at low speed just until combined. Add milk mixture; mix just until combined. Add remaining flour mixture; mix until combined. Stir in zucchini and chocolate chips.

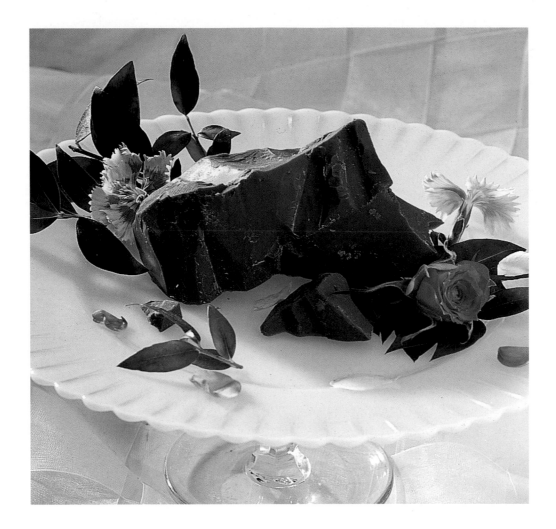

④ Spoon batter into pan. Bake 55 to 60 minutes or until top feels firm to touch and toothpick inserted in center comes out clean. Cool in pan on wire rack 15 minutes. Invert onto rack; cool completely.

⑤ In double broiler over barely simmering water, melt chocolate and orange juice. Stir until smooth. Drizzle over top and sides of cake.

12 servings.
Preparation time: 30 minutes. Ready to serve: 3 hours, 40 minutes.

Per serving: 460 calories, 20 g total fat (12 g saturated fat), 85 mg cholesterol, 360 mg sodium, 3.5 g fiber.

GREEN TOMATO PIE

This is an old-fashioned dessert designed to use up green tomatoes at season's end. Its resemblance to classic apple pie is uncanny.

CRUST

2¼	cups all-purpose flour
½	teaspoon salt
¾	cup unsalted butter, cut into ½-inch cubes
2	tablespoons shortening or unsalted butter
5 to 6	tablespoons ice water

FILLING

4	cups green tomatoes, sliced ¼- to ½-inch thick
2	cups peeled apples, sliced ¼- to ½-inch thick
1	teaspoon grated lime peel
1	cup sugar
¼	cup all-purpose flour
1	teaspoon ground cinnamon

❶ Combine 2¼ cups flour and ½ teaspoon salt in medium mixing bowl. Add butter and shortening; toss to coat. Work with pastry blender or 2 knives, work butter and shortening into flour until mixture resembles coarse meal with some larger pieces of butter remaining. Toss with just enough water to form a ball. Divide dough into 2 pieces; roll each into a ball, one slightly larger than the other. Shape dough into flat disk; wrap in plastic wrap. Refrigerate 1 hour.

❷ Heat oven to 425°F. Combine tomatoes, apples and lime peel in large mixing bowl. In small bowl, stir together sugar, ¼ cup flour and cinnamon. Toss with apple mixture.

❸ Roll out larger disk of dough to ⅛-inch thickness. Line 9-inch pie pan with dough. Fill with apple mixture. Roll out small disk of dough to ⅛-inch thickness; place over apple mixture. Pinch edges of crust together to seal; trim overhang. Cut slits in top to allow steam to escape.

❹ Bake at 425°F for 15 minutes. Reduce oven temperature to 375°F; continue baking an additional 40 to 50 minutes or until juices are bubbly. If pie crust appears to be browning too quickly, cover edges with foil to protect crust.

8 servings.
Preparation time: 30 minutes. Ready to serve: 4 hours.

Per serving: 455 calories, 21 g total fat (11.5 g saturated fat), 45 mg cholesterol, 155 mg sodium, 2.5 g fiber.

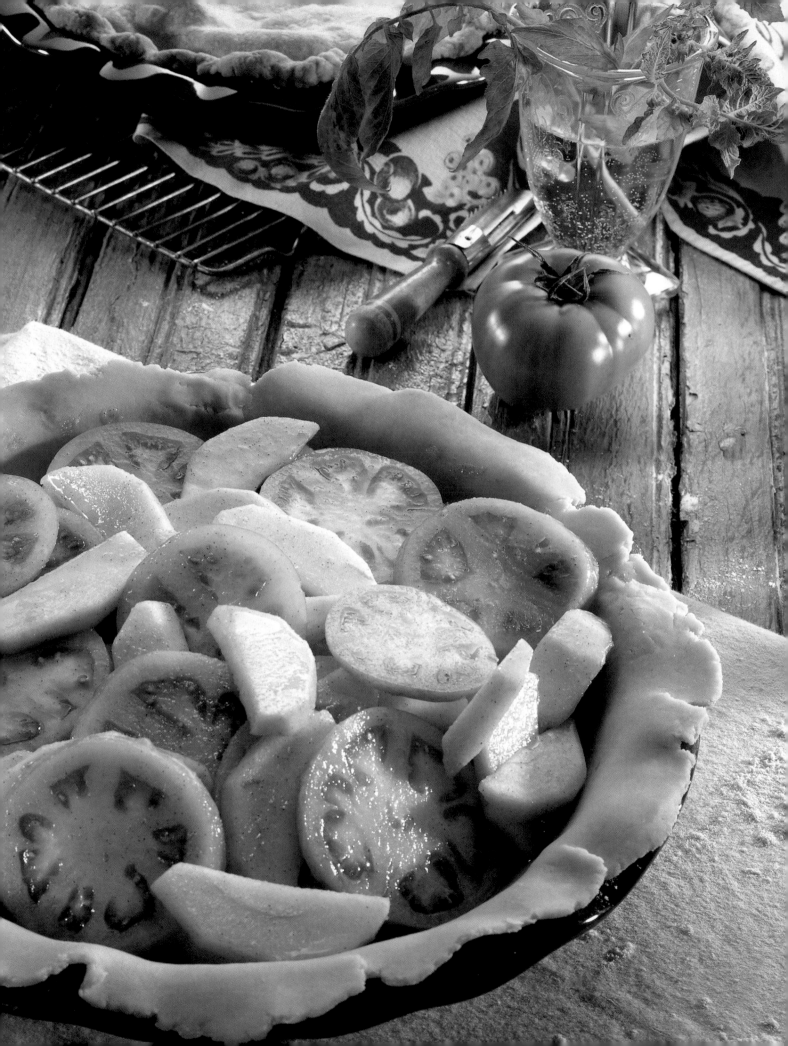

APPLE AND WALNUT CAKE WITH CARAMEL SAUCE

Beets add sweetness and color to this moist fall cake.

CAKE
- 1/2 cup unsalted butter, softened
- 1 3/4 cups plus 1/3 cup sugar
- 3 eggs
- 1 1/2 cups unsweetened applesauce
- 3 cups all-purpose flour
- 1 1/2 teaspoons baking soda
- 2 1/2 teaspoons ground cinnamon
- 1 teaspoon salt
- 1/2 teaspoon ground nutmeg
- 1/2 teaspoon ground allspice
- 1 medium Granny Smith apple, peeled, chopped (about 1 cup)
- 1 beet, cooked, peeled, cut into 1/4-inch pieces (about 1 cup)
- 1/2 cup chopped walnuts

SAUCE
- 1/2 cup unsalted butter
- 1 1/2 cups packed light brown sugar
- 1 cup heavy cream

1. Heat oven to 350°F. Grease and flour a 13 x 9-inch pan. Beat 1/2 cup butter in large mixer bowl at medium speed until creamy. Add 1 3/4 cups sugar and beat until fluffy. Add eggs one at a time, beating well after each addition. Mixture will look curdled. Stir in applesauce.

2. In large bowl, sift together flour, baking soda, 1 1/2 teaspoons of the cinnamon, salt, nutmeg and allspice. Add to applesauce mixture; beat at low speed until combined. Increase speed to medium; beat 30 seconds. Stir in apples, beets and walnuts. Spread into pan.

3. In small bowl, combine remaining 1/3 cup sugar and 1 teaspoon cinnamon; sprinkle over surface of cake. Bake 60 to 65 minutes or until toothpick inserted in center comes out clean. Cool on wire rack.

4. In medium saucepan, melt 1/2 cup butter over medium heat until medium brown in color. Add brown sugar and cream; bring to a boil, stirring constantly. Boil 1 minute. Remove from heat; cool slightly.

5. Place pool of caramel sauce on each plate; top with piece of cake.

15 servings.
Preparation time: 30 minutes. Ready to serve: 4 hours, 30 minutes.
Per serving: 495 calories, 21 g total fat (11.5 g saturated fat), 95 mg cholesterol, 315 mg sodium, 1.5 g fiber.

CARROT AND CARDAMOM COOKIES

Cardamom and almond are traditional Scandinavian flavorings. Here they team up with orange flecks of carrot and green pistachios for great taste and visual appeal.

1/2 cup butter
1 cup sugar
1 cup packed brown sugar
2 eggs
1/2 teaspoon almond extract
3 1/4 cups all-purpose flour
2 teaspoons ground cardamom
1 teaspoon baking soda
1/4 teaspoon salt
1 cup shredded carrots
1/2 cup chopped pistachios

❶ Heat oven to 375°F. Line baking sheet with parchment paper. In large bowl, beat butter, sugar and brown sugar at medium speed until well combined. Add eggs 1 at a time, beating well after each addition. Add almond extract; mix well. In another large bowl, sift together flour, cardamom, baking soda and salt. Add to butter mixture; beat at low speed just until combined. Stir in carrots and pistachios.

❷ Form dough into 1-inch balls. Place on baking sheet. Flatten with tines of fork dipped in sugar. Bake 9 to 11 minutes or until lightly browned. Cool on wire racks. Store in tightly covered containers.

5 dozen cookies.
Preparation time: 45 minutes. Ready to serve: 1 hour, 30 minutes.
Per cookie: 75 calories, 2.5 g total fat (1 g saturated fat), 10 mg cholesterol, 45 mg sodium, .5 g fiber.

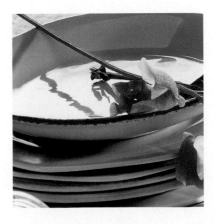

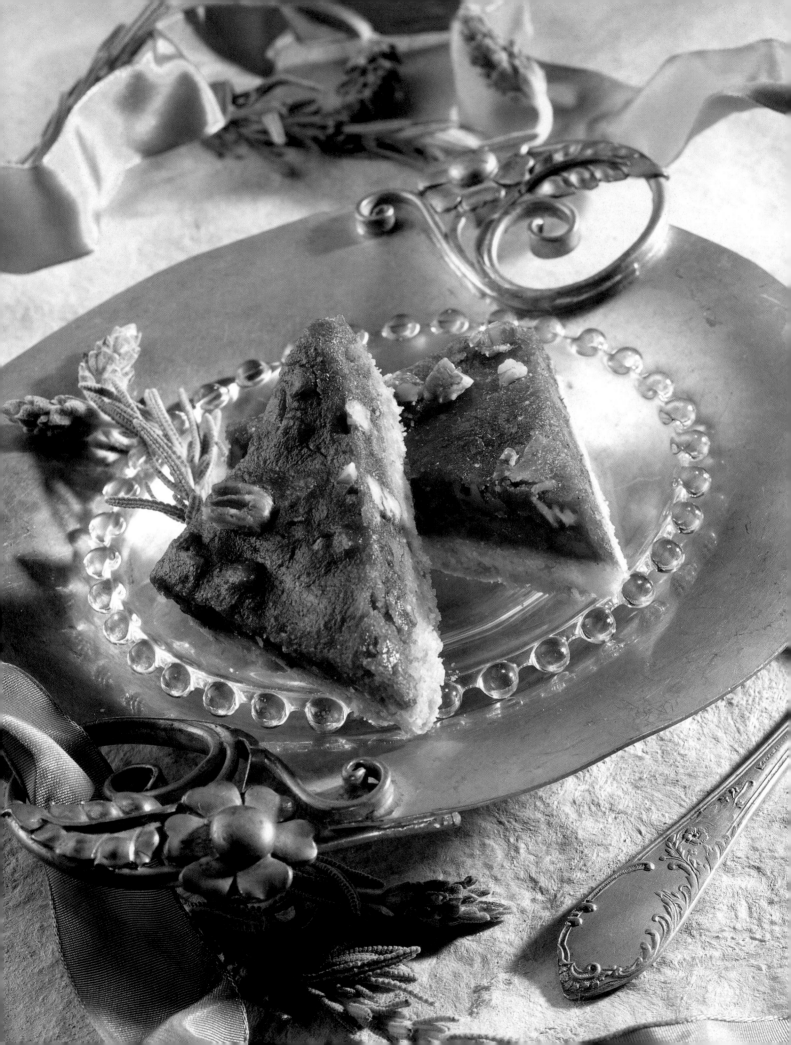

PUMPKIN-PECAN BARS

A cross between pumpkin and pecan pie, these bars are great to bake-and-take.

1 3/4   cups all-purpose flour
  3/4   cup butter
  1/3   cup powdered sugar
    2   cups cooked pumpkin* (or 1 (15-oz.) can)
    1   cup sugar
    1   cup dark corn syrup
    3   eggs
    2   tablespoons butter, melted, cooled
    1   teaspoon vanilla
  1/2   teaspoon ground cinnamon
  1/4   teaspoon salt
1 1/2   cups chopped pecans

❶ Heat oven to 350°F. In food processor, pulse together 1 1/2 cups of the flour, butter and powdered sugar. (Mixture will be dry.) Place mixture in 13 x 9-inch pan; press into bottom of pan. Bake 15 minutes or until lightly browned.

❷ In food processor, combine pumpkin and sugar; pulse to combine. Pulse in corn syrup, eggs, butter and vanilla. In small bowl, combine together 1/4 cup flour, cinnamon and salt. Pulse just until combined. Stir in pecans. Pour over crust. Bake 55 to 60 minutes or until top is no longer sticky to the touch. Cool on wire rack.

TIP *See *Maple-Pumpkin Cheesecake* (page 126) for directions on cooking pumpkin.

48 bars.
Preparation time: 10 minutes. Ready to serve: 4 hours.
Per bar: 120 calories, 6.5 g total fat (2.5 g saturated fat), 20 mg cholesterol, 45 mg sodium, 1 g fiber.

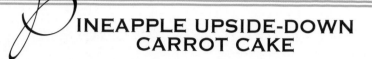

PINEAPPLE UPSIDE-DOWN CARROT CAKE

This recipe combines two traditional American favorites — pineapple upside-down cake and carrot cake — into one fabulous dessert.

6	tablespoons butter, melted
1½	cups packed brown sugar
3	(8-oz.) cans pineapple slices, drained
12	maraschino cherries
1¾	cups sugar
1	cup vegetable oil
2	teaspoons vanilla
3	eggs
2½	cups all-purpose flour
2	teaspoons baking soda
1	teaspoon ground cinnamon
¾	teaspoon salt
½	teaspoon ground ginger
2½	cups shredded carrots

❶ Heat oven to 350°F. Pour butter into 13 x 9-inch pan, brushing bottom and sides with butter. Sprinkle brown sugar evenly over bottom of pan; top with pineapple slices. Place maraschino cherry in center of each pineapple slice.

❷ In large bowl, combine sugar, oil, vanilla and eggs; beat well. In another large bowl, sift together flour, baking soda, cinnamon, salt and ginger. Add flour mixture to sugar mixture; mix well. Stir in carrots.

❸ Pour batter into pan. Bake 55 to 60 minutes or until cake springs back when lightly touched in center. Cool on wire rack 5 minutes. Invert onto serving platter; cool completely.

12 servings.
Preparation time: 20 minutes. Ready to serve: 3 hours, 20 minutes.
Per serving: 580 calories, 25.5 g total fat (6.5 g saturated fat), 70 mg cholesterol, 430 mg sodium, 2 g fiber.

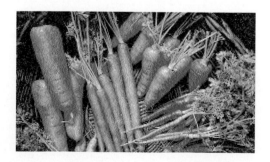

SQUASH GINGERBREAD

The squash adds moistness and flavor to this cold-weather favorite. Serve it with hot caramel sauce or with a scoop of vanilla ice cream.

1/2	cup pureed cooked squash*
1/2	cup packed light brown sugar
1/3	cup vegetable oil
1	egg
1/2	cup light molasses
1/2	cup water
1 1/2	cups all-purpose flour
1 1/4	teaspoons ground ginger
1	teaspoon baking powder
1/2	teaspoon baking soda
1/2	teaspoon ground cinnamon
1/4	teaspoon salt
1/4	teaspoon ground cloves

1 Heat oven to 350°F. Grease bottom of 8-inch square pan. In medium bowl, beat together squash, brown sugar and oil. Beat in egg, molasses and water. In another medium bowl, sift together flour, ginger, baking powder, baking soda, cinnamon, salt and cloves. Add flour mixture to squash mixture; mix.

2 Pour into pan. Bake 40 to 45 minutes or until top is firm and toothpick inserted in center comes out clean.

TIP *See *Squash Ravioli with Red Pepper Sauce* (page 112) for instructions on cooking squash.

9 servings.
Preparation time: 10 minutes. Ready to serve: 3 hours.
Per serving: 255 calories, 9 g total fat (1.5 g saturated fat), 25 mg cholesterol, 210 mg sodium, 1 g fiber.

SWEET POTATO CREME BRULEE

Brown sugar is the best sugar choice for making crème brûlée under the broiler. If you own a small torch, sold in specialty cookware stores, substitute granulated sugar instead and follow manufacturer's directions to use the torch.

1	cup cooked sweet potato*
1/2	cup sugar
2	cups half-and-half
4	egg yolks
2	eggs
2	tablespoons orange liqueur
1	tablespoon finely grated orange peel
1/4	teaspoon ground nutmeg
1/4	cup packed brown sugar

1 Heat oven to 350°F. Place sweet potato and sugar in food processor; pulse to form a smooth puree, scraping sides as necessary. Pulse in half-and-half just until combined; pulse in egg yolks and eggs just until combined. Strain into large bowl.

2 Stir in orange liqueur, orange peel and nutmeg. Pour into 6 (6-oz.) custard cups; place in 13 x 9-inch pan. Add enough boiling water to pan to come halfway up sides of custard cups. Bake 30 to 35 minutes or until centers are just set. Cool on wire rack 30 minutes. Refrigerate several hours or overnight.

3 Before serving, heat broiler. Press 2 teaspoons brown sugar through strainer over surface of each custard cup. Spread to evenly cover surface. Place custard cups in shallow pan; broil approximately 2 minutes or until brown sugar has melted. (Crème brûlée can be caramelized up to 2 hours ahead; cover and refrigerate.)

TIP *To cook sweet potato, place on baking sheet; cook at 400°F for 1 hour or until flesh is soft.

6 servings.
Preparation time: 25 minutes. Ready to serve: 4 hours, 10 minutes.
Per serving: 320 calories, 14.5 g total fat (7.5 g saturated fat), 240 mg cholesterol, 65 mg sodium, .5 g fiber.

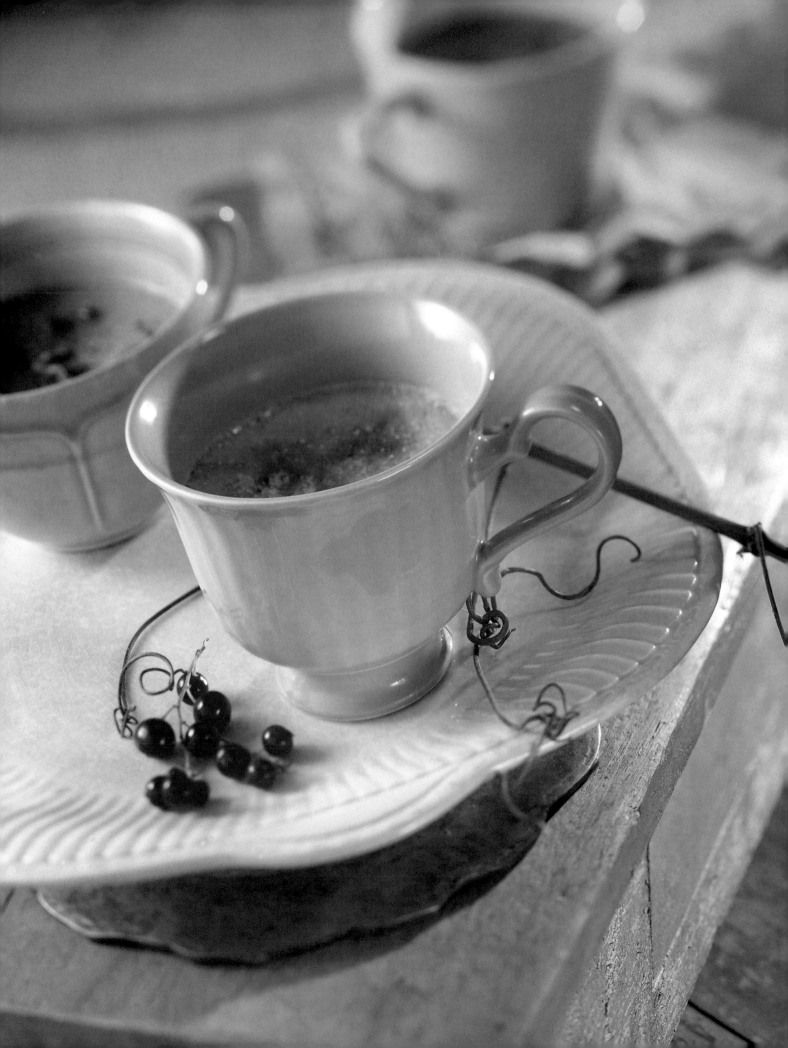

GLOSSARY

ARTICHOKES: A member of the thistle family, artichokes are at their peak in spring. California is our biggest producer. Available in many forms, baby artichokes are eaten whole. For mature artichokes, the edible portions are its heart, bottom and the base of its leaves. Look for unblemished, heavy artichokes with tight leaves. Refrigerate, unwashed, in a plastic bag for several days. Frozen or canned artichoke hearts or bottoms make acceptable substitutions. One cooked artichoke contains 531 mg vitamin A, .33 mg vitamin B-6, 30 mg vitamin C, 153 mg folic acid, 135 mg calcium and 3.87 mg iron.

ASPARAGUS: A member of the lily family, asparagus is a spring vegetable. It is usually found as green spears or sometimes purple, although European asparagus is often white. Early asparagus is pencil-thin but appears later with thicker spears. Look for smooth, firm stalks and closed, tight tips. Store in the refrigerator upright in an inch or two of water, covered in plastic or simply wrapped airtight, for several days. Best fresh. One half-cup of cooked, fresh asparagus contains 485 mg vitamin A, .11 mg vitamin B-6, 10 mg of vitamin C and 131 mg folic acid.

BEANS: Also called legumes, beans are grown and consumed worldwide and are a summer and fall vegetable. Consisting of a pod and inner seed, legume varieties consumed as pod and seed include

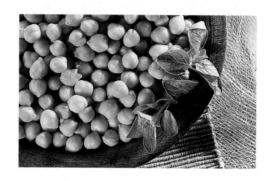

green and **yellow snap beans. Lima beans** are one of the fresh varieties consumed by eating just the seed. Dried (sometimes sold cooked and canned) varieties include **black, cannellini, chickpeas** or **garbanzo beans, Great Northern, kidney, navy, red and soy.** In fresh green and yellow beans, look for long, slender, firm, unblemished pods. Lima beans should be firm and unblemished. Store fresh beans in the refrigerator, airtight, for four to five days. Frozen green, yellow and lima beans make acceptable substitutions. One-half cup cooked, fresh green and yellow beans contains 413 mg vitamin A. One-half cup cooked lima beans contains 2.2 mg iron. Dried beans are a good source of protein.

BEETS: See root vegetables

BOK CHOY: See cabbages

BROCCOLI: A cruciferous vegetable, broccoli is related to the cabbage. Popular since Roman times, it is a cool-weather crop. Look for tight buds and firm stems. Avoid any sign of yellowing tips or woody stalks. Store in the refrigerator, airtight, for several days. Best fresh, but frozen broccoli is acceptable for cooking. One-half cup of broccoli contains 108 mg vitamin A, .11 mg vitamin B-6, 58 mg vitamin C and 36 mg calcium.

CABBAGES: Members of the *Brassica* family, the many types

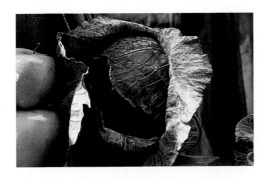

of cabbages are cruciferous vegetables. They come into their own in cooler weather. The most commonly found variety in this country has tight **green** or **red**

leaves shaped in a round head. Other varieties include Asian **bok choy**, which has firm, white stalks and dark green leaves; and **Napa cabbage,** which has an oblong shape and crinkly, pale leaves with lighter centers. **Savoy cabbage** has a slightly rounded, looser head of crinkly leaves. All varieties should be crisp with no signs of wilting or blemishes and heavy for their size. Cabbages will keep in the refrigerator wrapped airtight for several days. The rounder heads will keep up to a week. Best fresh or preserved, as in sauerkraut or kimchee. One-half cup of cooked green cabbage has 99 mg vitamin A and 15 mg vitamin C; red cabbage contributes minimal amounts of vitamins. One-half cup of cooked bok choy contains 2183 mg vitamin A, .14 mg vitamin B-6, 22 mg vitamin C, 35 mg folic acid and 79 mg calcium. One-half cup cooked Napa cabbage contains 575 mg vitamin A, 9 mg vitamin C and 32 mg folic acid; one-half cup cooked Savoy cabbage has 649 mg vitamin A, 12 mg vitamin C and 34 mg folic acid.

CARROTS: See root vegetables

CAULIFLOWER: Another cruciferous vegetable, cauliflower grows best in cooler weather. The most common variety is white, but it can be found in green and purple varieties also. Look for firm, heavy bunches with no sign of browning. Refrigerate in a plastic bag with as little air as possible for several days. Frozen cauliflower is acceptable in cooking. One-half cup of cooked cauliflower contains 27 mg vitamin C and 27 mg folic acid.

CELERY: Originally a fall vegetable, celery is now available every season. Its most common variety is **Pascal** celery, found in bunched, firm, crisp ribs topped with tender leaves. Its close relative, **celery root** or **celeraic,** is a popular winter vegetable in Europe with a more intense celery flavor. Celery root has a knobby, round, brown-skinned exterior that, once peeled, exposes a pale, crisp, ivory interior. Pascal celery should be firm when purchased, with crisp, unblemished ribs. Its leaves should not be limp. Celery root should be small and firm, with as few knobs as possible. Refrigerate celery and celery root, stored in a plastic bag — celery for two weeks, celery root for one. Best fresh. One-half cup cooked celery contains 99 mg vitamin A and 66 mg calcium. Raw celery root (3.5-oz.) contributes 110 mg calcium to the diet.

CORN: A New World discovery, **sweet corn** is still far more popular here for eating than anywhere else. The essence of summer, corn has an endless variety of hybrids, appearing in yellow, white and a blend of both on the cob. Asian recipes call for **baby corn,** consisting of immature ears of sweet corn. Buy and eat as soon as possible after picking. The green leaves covering the ears should not be dry, the silk should not be withered, the kernels should extend to the top of the ear and moisture should spurt from the kernels when pierced. Keep refrigerated no more than a day. Frozen or canned corn is an acceptable substitution. One-half cup cooked corn contains 178 mg vitamin A.

CUCUMBERS: This ancient vegetable is a member of the gourd family. Available in various sizes, the longest is the **English cucumber,** a variety without seeds

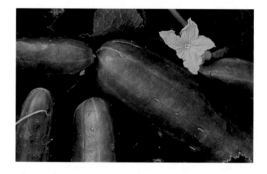

that grows up to two feet. Look for firm, smooth cucumbers. Smaller cucumbers tend to have smaller, less bitter seeds. Avoid any softness or withering. Refrigerate, wrapped in plastic, up to a week and a half. Best fresh or pickled. One-half cup raw cucumber contains 112 mg vitamin A.

EGGPLANT: A member of the nightshade family, this late summer vegetable is really a fruit. The most common eggplant is the large, teardrop-shaped variety with creamy flesh and a deep purple skin. **Japanese eggplant** is much smaller and narrower. **White eggplant** is egg-shaped and gives this vegetable its name. Asian markets feature a wide selection of different green varieties, some as small as cherries. Look for shiny, heavy, firm-skinned eggplants with no soft spots. Store at cool room temperature for a day or so or a bit longer stored in the refrigerator's vegetable crisper. Best fresh. Eggplant contributes minimal vitamins.

FENNEL: A cool-weather vegetable, fennel is primarily grown here and in the Mediterranean. Its most common variety, **Florence fennel,** has celery-like stems with feathery fronds and a broad base. The other variety, **common fennel,** produces fennel seeds. Fennel should be firm and crisp with no brown spots. Store refrigerated, wrapped airtight, for four to five days. Best fresh. One-half cup raw fennel contains 58 mg vitamin A and 22 mg calcium.

GARLIC: A member of the lily family, garlic is an early summer crop grown primarily in this country in California, Texas and Louisiana. Garlic comes with both white and purple skins or as **elephant garlic** with larger cloves and milder flavor. Some markets also offer **green garlic,** which is the immature shoot of the garlic plant before cloves are formed. Store at cool room temperature with air circulation. Available fresh, chopped or minced in refrigerated jars, or dehydrated. While low in vitamins and

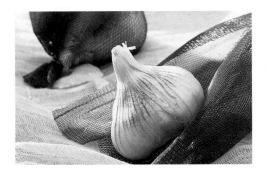

minerals, garlic has been attributed with healthful properties for centuries.

GREENS: A broad category of vegetable comprising the edible leaves of plants. A cool-weather crop, varieties include **collard, kale, mustard** and **spinach.** Look for fresh leaves, full of moisture, with no yellowing. Smaller leaves will be more tender. Store airtight in the refrigerator for several days. Best fresh, but frozen spinach works well in cooking. One-half cup cooked collard greens contains 1746 mg vitamin A and 15 mg calcium. One-half cup cooked kale contains 4810 mg vitamin A, 27 mg vitamin C and 31 mg calcium.

One-half cup cooked mustard greens contain 2122 mg vitamin A, 18 mg vitamin C, 51 mg folic acid and 52 mg calcium. One-half cup cooked spinach contains 7371 mg vitamin A, 9 mg vitamin C, .22 mg vitamin B-6, 131 mg folic acid and 122 mg calcium.

LEEKS: Related to the lily, leeks resemble an overgrown green onion with a white, slightly bulbous base and green, leafy top. A favorite in the Mediterranean, leeks favor the cooler months for growing. Look for small, firm, unblemished leeks with crisp-looking stems. Refrigerate loosely wrapped in a plastic bag for four to five days. Best fresh. Leeks contribute minimal vitamins.

LETTUCES: Primarily a cool-weather crop, these leafy vegetables include **Belgian endive, escarole, iceberg, leaf** and **romaine.** Belgian endive is a small, pale, oval head of tightly packed leaves with a slightly bitter flavor. Escarole is part of the same family, with broad leaves in a flatter head; its flavor is milder than Belgian endive. Iceberg lettuce comes in round heads of tightly packed, crunchy leaves with a neutral flavor. Leaf lettuces come in a variety of shapes and color tones, including red-tinted, distinguished by growing from a central stem into a loose bunch. Romaine grows in an elongated bunch, with

crunchy leaves that vary from dark green outside to pale inside. All lettuces should look fresh; avoid limp leaves with brown edges. Refrigerate lettuce, wrapped in a barely damp paper towel, in an airtight plastic bag for several days to a week depending on the variety. Best fresh. Belgian endive and iceberg lettuce contribute minimal vitamins; one-half cup escarole contains 99 mg folic acid and 90 mg calcium. One-half cup leaf lettuce contains 532 mg vitamin A; one-half cup romaine contains 728 mg vitamin A.

MUSHROOMS: This broad category of edible fungi has been grown for consumption since the Greeks and Romans. White mushrooms are cultivated year-round while exotic, or wild, mushrooms appear at different seasons throughout the year depending on the variety. Many

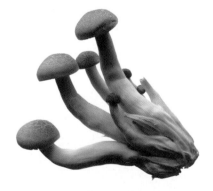

are now under cultivation, making them more accessible. The *Boletus* family of mushrooms is variously called **cèpes, porcini** and **steinpilze** depending on their country of origin. They are widely used in European cooking and are primarily available dried in this country. **Chanterelles** are trumpet-shaped mushrooms whose colors range from golden to orange. They are grown in Europe, the Pacific Northwest and the East Coast. **Portobello** mushrooms are larger versions of the cultivated **crimini** or brown mushroom. Fresh mushrooms should be unbroken and free of moist or discolored spots. Store them in the refrigerator, loosely covered, to allow for air circulation, for several days. Best fresh or dried but canned or frozen may be substituted. Mushrooms contribute minimal vitamins but are a satisfying, low-calorie and fat-free substitute for meat.

OKRA: Popular in the southern United States and in other hot climates, okra is a warm-weather crop. Tapered at one end, okra has ridged sides and an oblong shape. Look for firm, blemish-free pods. Avoid larger, woody pods; the smaller the pod, the more tender it will be. Refrigerate for several days in a plastic bag. Best fresh but frozen is an acceptable substitute in some recipes. One half cup cooked okra contains 411 mg vitamin A, 10 mg vitamin C, 116 mg folic acid and 77 mg calcium.

ONIONS: Related to lilies, this category includes **pearl onions, red onions, scallions** or **green onions** along with the more familiar **yellow** and **white onions.** Depending on the variety, their season extends from spring through the fall months and into winter. Green onions or scallions are harvested immaturely before the base has turned into the familiar large bulb of the dried onion. Pearl onions are small

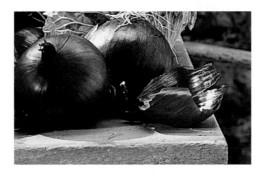

versions of the larger varieties. Other types include the **Bermuda, Globe, Maui, Spanish, Vidalia** and **Walla Walla onions** with flavors ranging from sweet to sharp. Yellow onions found in supermarkets are often the Bermuda or Spanish with relatively mild flavors. White onions have a silvery skin and are usually quite mild. Fresh, green onions should be crisp; dried onions should be firm. Avoid any with soft spots or molding. Store at cool room temperature with air circulation. Best fresh; some varieties are also available frozen or canned. One-half cup raw green onion contains 193 mg vitamin A and 36 mg calcium; the remainder contribute minimal vitamins.

PARSNIPS: See root vegetables

PEAS: A spring crop, peas are legumes. Their varieties include **English peas** which are normally eaten with shell removed, **sugar snap peas** which are eaten with both pod and pea, and **snow peas** or **pea pods** which are eaten for the pod. Look for fresh, crisp pods with no sign of wilting or spots. The inner pea should be smallish or, in the case of pea pods, virtually nonexistent. Best fresh but frozen may be substituted. One-half cup cooked, shelled peas contains 478 mg vitamin A, .18 mg vitamin B-6, 12 mg vitamin C, 51 mg folic acid and 22 mg calcium; one-half cup cooked edible pod peas contains 105 mg vitamin A, .12 mg vitamin B-6, 39 mg vitamin C and 34 mg calcium.

PEPPERS, SWEET AND HOT: These members of the *Capsicum* family range in flavor from sweet to hot and are a midsummer to early fall crop. Native to the Western Hemisphere, they are used globally. **Bell peppers,** so named because of their shape, start out green; some then ripen to red, yellow, orange and purple. Hot peppers are more often called chiles and come in a wide range of shapes, sizes and colors. Their heat comes from the seeds and membranes. Smaller chiles are often hotter. The Scoville scale rates the hotness of the pepper by determining the amount of capsaicin the pepper contains. **Anaheim peppers,** also called **New Mexico peppers,** are fairly mild, **jalapeño, chipotle** (smoked jalapeño) and **serrano peppers** are medium-hot. Bottled hot sauce is made from very hot peppers such as **habañero** or **tabasco.** (Names of chiles can vary depending on the regional cuisine, and some change names when dried, so ask questions if in doubt.) Look for

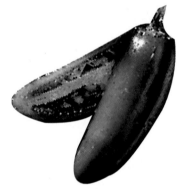

firm, heavy, blemish-free peppers with shiny skins. Refrigerate for up to a week in a plastic bag. One-half cup green sweet peppers contains 316 mg vitamin A, .12 mg vitamin B-6 and 45 mg vitamin C. Red sweet peppers contain 2850 mg vitamin A and 95 mg vitamin C. One hot pepper contains 347 mg vitamin A, .13 mg vitamin B-6 and 109 mg vitamin C. Red varieties contain 4838 mg vitamin A.

POTATOES: Being a member of the nightshade family, potatoes were once thought to be poisonous. Small, immature new potatoes are harvested in the spring and early summer with other varieties available year-round. **Idaho russets** are low in moisture and high in starch, giving them a fluffy texture when cooked. Moist **Yukon Golds** have a buttery color and **red** or **boiling potatoes** have a waxy, moist flesh that is low in starch. Potatoes should be firm, without spots, sprouts or greenish tinge. Store them at cool room temperature, away from light, for one to two weeks. Best fresh. One baked potato without skin contains .47 mg vitamin B-6 and 20 mg vitamin C. One boiled potato without skin contains .4 mg vitamin B-6 and 18 mg vitamin C.

PUMPKIN: See winter squashes

RADISHES: A member of the mustard family, radishes are a sign of spring but can be found year-round. Besides the familiar red, round radish, other varieties range in color from white to black. Shapes also vary such as the elongated, tapered oblong of the **daikon radish.** Radishes should be crisp and not yield when pressed. If sold with leaves attached, they should show no signs of wilting. Refrigerate for four to five days in a plastic bag. Best fresh. Radishes

contribute minimal vitamins.

ROOT VEGETABLES: So named because their edible portion grows beneath the ground, root vegetables are a mainstay of fall and winter cooking. **Beets,** also known as garden beets, are related to Swiss chard and sugar beets. Beets have a round, sweet base and crinkly leaves; both are edible. Besides the normal deep red, look

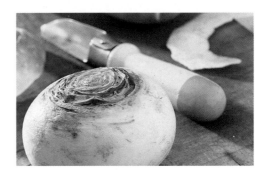

for yellow, white and **chioggia,** or candy cane, varieties. **Carrots** and **parsnips** are members of the parsley family and share a common sweetness of flavor. **Turnips** also have a mildly sweet flavor with a peppery finish. Look for firm root vegetables, never limp; the smaller vegetables are often more tender. Store beets trimmed of their greens. All root vegetables may be stored in the refrigerator in a plastic bag for up to two weeks. Beets may keep a bit longer, and turnips also store well at cool room temperature. All are best fresh. One-half cup cooked beets contains 68 mg folic acid and

These members of the Capsicum family range in flavor from sweet to hot and are a midsummer to early fall crop. Native to the Western Hemisphere, they are used globally. Bell peppers, so named because of their shape, start out green; some then ripen to red, yellow, orange and purple. Hot peppers are more often called chiles and come in a wide range of shapes, sizes and colors. Their heat comes from the seeds and membranes. Smaller chiles are often hotter. The Scoville scale rates the hotness of the pepper by determining the amount of capsaicin the pepper contains. Anaheim peppers, also called New Mexico peppers, are fairly mild, jalapeño, chipotle (smoked jalapeño) and serrano peppers are medium-hot. Bottled hot

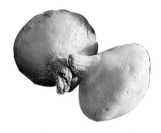

sauce is made from very hot peppers such as habañero or tabasco. (Names of chiles can vary depending on the regional cuisine, and some change names when dried, so ask questions if in doubt.) Look for firm, heavy, blemish-free peppers with shiny skins. Refrigerate for up to a week in a plastic bag. One-half cup green sweet peppers contains 316 mg vitamin A, .12 mg vitamin B-6 and 45 mg vitamin C. Red sweet peppers contain 2850 mg vitamin A and 95 mg vitamin C. One hot pepper contains 347 mg vitamin A, .13 mg vitamin B-6 and 109 mg vitamin C. Red varieties contain 4838 mg vitamin A.

POTATOES: Being a member of the nightshade family, potatoes were once thought to be poisonous. Small, immature new potatoes are harvested in the spring and early summer with other varieties available year-round. Idaho russets are low in moisture and high in starch, giving them a fluffy texture when cooked. Moist Yukon Golds have a buttery color and red or boiling potatoes have a waxy, moist flesh that is low in starch. Potatoes should be firm, without spots, sprouts or greenish tinge. Store them at cool room temperature, away from light, for one to two weeks. Best fresh. One baked potato was originally feared to be poisonous. Tomatoes come in an amazing variety of shapes and colors, ranging from vivid red globes to yellow pear shapes, with a full spectrum in between including green-striped and purple. The most common varieties include the round **beefsteak tomato** that's perfect for slicing, the pear-shaped **Roma** or **plum tomato** with lots of flesh and fewer seeds and the tiny **cherry tomato** used in salads or with dips. Look for heirloom

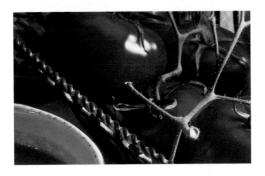

varieties grown from heritage seeds that have not been hybridized. Tomatoes should be heavy and slightly yielding with good color. Store at room temperature for several days. Best fresh or canned when out of season. One-half cup of cooked tomatoes contains 892 mg vitamin A, .11 mg vitamin B-6 and 27 mg vitamin C.

WINTER SQUASHES: These members of the gourd family have harder skins and seeds than their summer cousins, and come into their own in the fall and winter. Common varieties include **acorn**

squash, shaped like its namesake with a green skin, and **butternut squash** with a narrower neck, bulbous base and pale, slightly rosy-beige skin. **Hubbard squash** are large and bumpy while **spaghetti squash** have yellow skins with pasta-like flesh. **Pumpkins,** a mainstay of the early Colonial diet, are known for their round, orange exterior. Smaller pumpkins are tastier than their larger varieties. All winter squash should be heavy and blemish-free with hard exteriors. Store at cool room temperature in a dark place. Squash are available fresh, frozen or canned. One-half cup baked acorn squash contains 437 mg vitamin A, .2 mg vitamin B-6, 11 mg vitamin C and 12 mg calcium; one-half cup baked butternut squash contains 7141 mg vitamin A, .13 mg vitamin B-6, 115 mg vitamin C and 42 mg calcium. One-half cup cooked hubbard squash contains 4726 mg vitamin A, .12 mg vitamin B-6, 8 mg vitamin C and 12 mg calcium; one-half cup cooked spaghetti squash contains 86 mg vitamin A and 16 mg calcium. One-half cup of cooked pumpkin contains 1320 mg vitamin A and 18 mg calcium.

SOURCES

Here is a listing of possible mail order and Internet sources
for hard-to-find ingredients.

Adriana's Caravan
409 Vanderbilt Street
Brooklyn, NY 11218
1 (800) 316-0820

www.adrianascaravan.com

Source for international ingredients,
including North African

Joie de Vivre
P. O. Box 875
Modesto, CA 95353
1 (800) 648-8854

Source for French ingredients

Coyote Café General Store
132 West Water Street
Santa Fe, NM 87501
1 (800) 866-4695

www.coyotecafeatmgm.com

Source for southwestern ingredients

Pacific Island Market
4111 Mexico Road
St. Peters, MO 63376
1 (877) 274-2639

www.asiamex.com

Source for Asian and Mexican
ingredients

Dean and Deluca
560 Broadway
New York, NY 10012
1 (800) 221-7714

www.dean-deluca.com

Source for gourmet foods

Penzeys
P. O. Box 933
Muskego, WI 53150
1 (800) 741-7787

www.penzeys.com

Source for spices and herbs

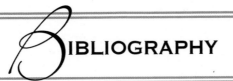

BIBLIOGRAPHY

These materials have been a source of inspiration and information in writing this book.

Fletcher, Janet. *Fresh from the Farmers' Market.* San Francisco: Chronicle Books, 1997.

Greene, Bert. *Greene on Greens.* New York: Workman Publishing, 1984.

Herbst, Sharon Tyler. *The New Food Lover's Companion.* New York: Barrons, 1995.

Madison, Deborah. *Vegetarian Cooking for Everyone.* New York: Broadway Books, 1997.

Pennington, Jean A. *Bowes and Church's Food Values of Portions Commonly Used.* Philadelphia: Lippincott, 1998.

Sinclair, Charles. *International Dictionary of Food and Cooking.* Great Britain: Peter Collin Publishing, 1998.

RECIPE INDEX

This index lists every recipe in Vegetable Creations *by name. If you're looking for a specific recipe but can't recall the exact name, refer to the General Index that starts on page 153.*

GENERAL INDEX

There are several ways to use this helpful index. First — you can find recipes by name. If you don't know a recipe's specific name but recall a main vegetable ingredient, look under that heading and all the recipes using that ingredient will be listed; scan for the recipe you want. If you have a vegetable in mind and want to find a great recipe for it, look under that ingredient heading as well to find a list of recipes to choose from. Finally — you can use this general index to find a summary of the recipes in each chapter of the book (appetizers, side dishes, salads, etc.).